Your HAIR
and
Your HEALTH

By PAUL C. BRAGG, N.D., Ph.D.

with

PATRICIA BRAGG Ph.D.

Health and Beauty Consultant

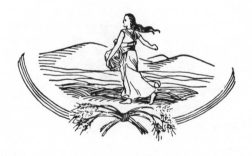

Published by

HEALTH SCIENCE

Box 7, Santa Barbara, California 93102 U.S.A.

YOUR HAIR AND YOUR HEALTH

Natural Method
of
Hair Improvement for Men and Women

By PAUL C. BRAGG, N.D., Ph.D.
with
PATRICIA BRAGG Ph.D.

Copyright © Health Science 1977

Twelfth Printing MCMLXXIX

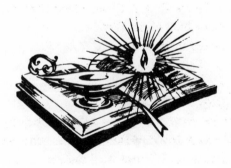

Published in the United States by
HEALTH SCIENCE - Box 7, Santa Barbara, California 93102, U.S.A.

Library of Congress Catalog Card Number: 68-24214
I S B N :   0-87790-009-4

PRINTED IN THE UNITED STATES OF AMERICA

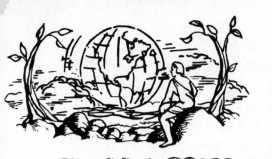

CONTENTS

Contents

Contents

The best service a book can render is, to impart truth, but to make you think it out for yourself.
—Elbert Hubbard

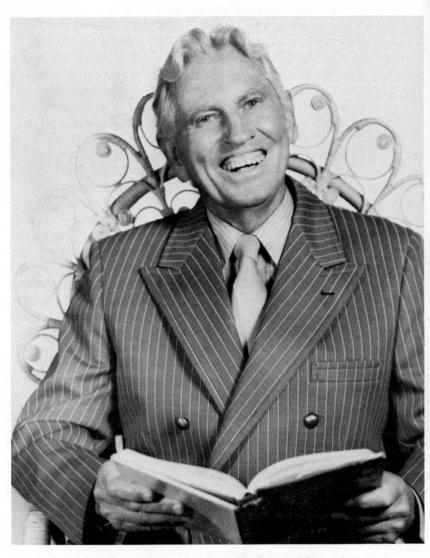

NATURE INTENDED YOUR HAIR TO BE
HEALTHY, THICK AND LUXURIANT!

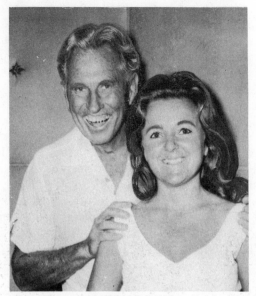

Paul E. Bragg and daughter Patricia

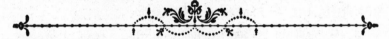

WHY WE WROTE THIS BOOK:

Traveling as we do throughout the English speaking world, lecturing on the subject of Nutrition and Physical Culture, we meet thousands of men and women with hair problems of all kinds.

In the United States alone there are 15,000,000 bald men. And these are not all old men ... some are under 20 years of age. It is a conservative estimate to say that 30,000,000 youths are headed toward baldness—unless something is done to prevent it.

True, not one woman in 20,000 is bald ... but there are thousands of women who are partially bald. Tens of thousands of others have unmanageable, stubby, thin, weak, unbecoming hair. There are thousands whose scalps are in poor condition causing constant scratching due to irritation and dandruff.

This book is not a cure for baldness or a cure for unhealthy scalp conditions. It is a book to tell you how to take care of your Hair and Scalp Health.

It will explain the causes of unhealthy hair and scalp conditions. It will give you a Natural Program for keeping the hair and scalp in perfect condition.

Any unusual condition of the scalp—such as excessive dryness, excessive oiliness, sudden falling out of the hair, excessive dandruff—is a signal from the body that something is wrong. As a matter of fact, it is most often a symptom of unhygienic living habits, wrong diet, autointoxication, poor circulation to hair and scalp, lack of sleep or excessive nerve strain which weakens the entire constitution.

This book will teach you how to return to Natural, Healthful Ways of Living. Good health promotes good healthy hair and scalp. That is the reason the title of this book is YOUR HAIR AND YOUR HEALTH.

INTRODUCTION

BEAUTIFUL HAIR—The Secret of Attraction

This remarkable book teaches you the correct, harmless NATURAL WAY to combat hair and scalp problems. Nature intended you to have healthy hair—thick and luxuriant —regardless of your age. Read this book and we are quite sure you will agree that it is one of—if not the—most valuable and instructive books ever written on Hair and Scalp Culture. Results are certain to be beneficial if instructions are properly followed.

Here is a penetrating study of a subject vitally important to the young and the mature alike.

You have often heard it remarked, "How beautiful she is!" ... or, "What a handsome man!" Yet have you ever stopped to consider what prompted the compliment? It was their "Crowning Glory" ... they had luxuriantly thick hair with that soft, glossy, well groomed appearance—healthy hair!

Within the pages of this book you will find a priceless Natural Program to Help YOU Attain Hair and Scalp Health.

—Paul C. Bragg and Patricia Bragg

YOUR HEALTH AND YOUR HAIR
The Bragg Natural Method
of
Hair Improvement

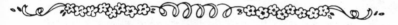

**NATURE INTENDED YOUR HAIR TO BE
HEALTHY, THICK AND LUXURIANT!**

It is your birthright to have a full head of healthy hair regardless of your age! Nature intended your hair to be beautiful and plentiful. There is no age limit. Everyone—from infants to great-grandparents—should have thick, strong, goodlooking hair. Nature provided everything to make it so. But 'many people have never knôwn naturally thick, strong, healthy hair ... simply because they do not know how to take care of the hair and scalp.

MOST PEOPLE HAVE A HAIR PROBLEM OF SOME KIND

We see people with thin, weak, fragile hair. We find a great deal of baldness. We meet people with dry hair or oily hair or unmanageable hair ... hair that looks like straw with no sheen or sparkle. We encounter people not only with problems of the hair ... but also with problems of the scalp—such as dandruff, scaly scalp, itchy scalp, tight scalp and many other poor scalp conditions.

No other part of the body engages quite so much daily attention as the hair and scalp. Everyone has hair ... often either too much or too little. And too late, usually, everyone becomes interested in his hair. Seldom is anyone completely satisfied with it.

Hair—is it a useful portion of the body ... or is it merely an inevitable appendage on which we spend so much time in combing, brushing, washing, cutting and arranging and talking about?

Our hair is of great importance in our lives. It is called our "Crowning Glory"—and it can make us either attractive or unattractive. That is why we have such a rapidly multiplying number of Hairdressing Establishments, Barber Shops and (of all things!) Men's Hair Styling Shops, all trying to help in making hair attractive and beautiful.

MYTHS AND MISINFORMATION ABOUT THE HAIR

For all its attention, this commonplace attribute—hair—attracts a surprising mass of delusions and contradictions. Most people know less about hair than about any other equally important part of the body. Many people believe that baldness and poor hair in general are due to heredity. I have had women say to me, "I take after my mother. She had thin, weak hair." ... and I have had men say to me, "My father started losing his hair when he was nineteen, and by the time he was twenty-five he was completely bald. I take after him."

Baldness and weak hair in both men and women (many women start getting bald very young in life) are said to be caused by anything from sleeping in short beds to wearing hats or not wearing hats. Many will tell you that frequent washing is bad for the hair. But in the South Sea Islands where both men and women have thick, beautiful hair, they spend hours upon hours in the water. Others will tell you to keep out of the sun or the sun will kill the hair root. Again let me say that the natives of the South Sea Islands expose their hair to the sunshine hours upon hours, and they are noted for their strong, beautiful hair.

Failing vision is not entrusted to makers of glass eyes, nor gouty feet to wooden-leg manufacturers. Yet we often stake our cherished heads of hair on the "profound" knowledge of people who believe that cut hair "bleeds" and must be singed lest it die ... and we pay any price asked for medicated soaps whose only virtue is in cleansing the scalp. People tend to

2

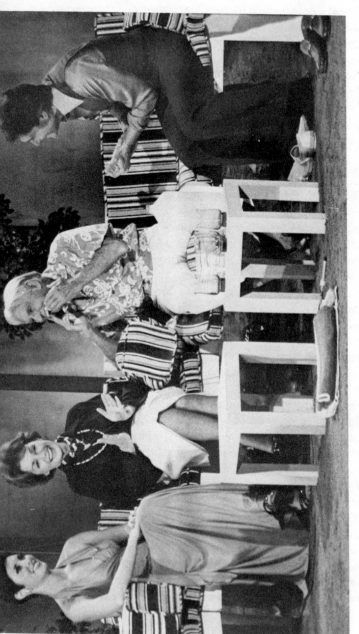

Paul Bragg and Lilly Palmer, famous English Actress were both guests on Hollywood's Beverly and Vidal Sasson T.V. Show. Vidal is the world famous hair-designer to the most glamorous women in the world and his show is geared towards keeping youthful and attractive. Above, Bragg shows that you can have all your own teeth like he has and a full head of healthy hair—How? By living a health life free from refined foods.

take more bad advice about the hair than about almost any other part of the body.

The readiness to believe so many myths and fables can only be ascribed to a faulty comprehension of the nature of hair itself ... otherwise, common sense would intervene. In the general misconceptions there are two chief factors:

First, the vague belief that hair is an independent product of the body, formed of a different substance—a sort of crop no more closely related to the body than grass to earth;

Second, the ill-defined feeling that hair has a life of its own.

LEARN THE TRUE FACTS ABOUT HAIR AND HEALTH

These erroneous ideas are at the root of most ignorance concerning hair, and their effect is graver than might seem. The belief that hair has a life of its own leads to the use of various hair preparations, lotions and tonics, and a consequent dependence on these ... to the neglect of the important bodily nutrition of the hair and scalp.

Preparations, lotions and tonics will not feed the hair. Hair is built by the blood stream. Hair is very much like the muscles of the body in growth and nourishment. To be strong and supple, the muscles must be fed correctly and exercised regularly. So should the hair. And that is what we are going to explain to you in this book: *How to keep your hair fit.*

If you are losing or have lost much of your hair, or if you are bald and want to regain at least some of it, you should do all in your power to build a healthy blood stream. I have absolutely no cures for baldness. Baldness may be due to some deficiency within the blood stream, or lack of circulation, etc.

Hair grows in a kind of body soil—and I don't mean dirt!— that is just under the scalp. When people have a rich, nourishing "hair soil" they have no hair or scalp problems. When this soil becomes depleted of essential nutrients, then the problems of the hair and scalp begin. The bald person loses the hair soil on top of the head. That is why you see men and women who are often bald on top of their heads, although they may have a very thick and healthy hair around the lower part of the head. This indicates that the soil has dropped from the top of the head to the lower part of the scalp.

YOUR HAIR AND YOUR BLOOD

In this book we are going to help you to help yourself toward better hair and scalp health. There are no miracle treatments that will grow hair on bald heads. But we are going to show you how to feed your blood stream so that you will have the required nutrients to feed the hair soil. We are going to teach you how to take good care of your hair by proper massage, brushing, shampooing and correct cleansing.

We want you to keep this in mind ... that the hair is as much a part of your body as are the nails and skin, and is formed of precisely the same substance, and is equally dependent upon the body for nourishment and life. Actually, the health of the body is reflected in the health of the hair.

Ill health usually results in an unhealthy condition of the hair. After long high fevers, for example, there will often be great loss of hair. The average sick person loses the sheen and vitality of the hair ... like the skin, it becomes dead-looking, and is usually unmanageable and unsightly.

Hair certainly reflects the condition of your general health. This is very obvious in animals. When an animal is sick, the fur becomes ugly and loses its shiny gloss. As soon as the animal gets well, the condition of the fur shows it at once.

So keep this in mind ... the better your health, the better the condition of your hair. It cannot be said too often that the way to keep hair healthy is to keep the body healthy ... and to do it in time, so as not to suffer loss of hair.

Understand that we are setting forth no claims of having discovered a cure for baldness. We do not believe in manmade cures. Only Mother Nature can cure.

We are interested in the causes of baldness and other unhealthy hair conditions. We believe that one of the main causes is a nutritional deficiency in the blood stream. If the hair soil is not fed, the hair either will not grow or will produce a poor crop of hair. Toxic poisons in the body have a great deal to do with killing the hair, or stifling it so that the hair is of poor quality.

There is also the condition produced by obstructing the circulation of the blood in the scalp over a prolonged period, and at certain well defined places on the head. Removing the obstruction is one of the first steps in the program, but that is not enough. Another step is to restore the cranial blood vessels to their natural, normal state and to maintain them in that condition.

Do not become discouraged because you have some kind of hair or scalp problem. Read this book through several times and apply its teachings.

WHAT HAIR IS AND WHAT IT DOES

A hair has three layers. The outer or horny layer is composed of smooth, flat, transparent cells piled upon one another like shingles on a roof. Because of this arrangement and the density of the cells, this outer layer forms a very effective shield for the inner part of the hair. It has been observed that the hair is the least destructible part of the body and the last of the human tissues to decay.

The second layer or cortex is composed of elongated cells which give the hair its flexibility. When these cells cease to function the hair breaks. Small openings in the cortex hold the oil which gives the hair its sheen. Lacking this oil, the hair appears dry, dull and harsh. The natural coloring matter is contained in this second layer, and shows through the outer layer to give the hair its tones of brown, red, black, yellow, gray or white. (The nature of this pigmentation will be discussed in more detail later when we go into the problem of gray hair.)

The central layer of the hair is the marrow canal or medulla, composed of two rows of cells placed side by side lengthwise of the shaft. It should be clearly realized that the medulla or marrow canal is not hollow. It forms the strong core of the hair. Weak hairs and the soft, colorless, downy hairs of the body lack this central core.

There is nothing more expensive than ignorance in action.

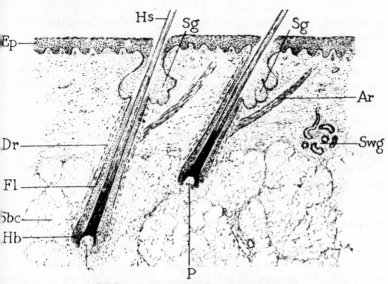

SECTION THROUGH THE SCALP

Ep—Epidermis
Hs—Hairshaft
Fl—Follicle
Dr—Dermal coat of the follicle.
Hb—Hair bulb

P—Papilla
Sg—Sebaceous gland
Swg—Sweat gland
Sbc—Subcutaneous tissue
Ar—Arrector pili muscle

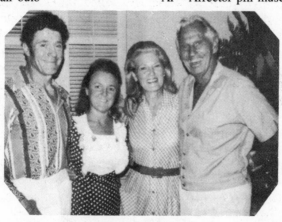

Jack LaLanne, Patricia Bragg, Elaine LaLanne & Paul Bragg

Jack says, "Bragg saved my life at age 14 when I attended the Bragg Health & Fitness Lecture in Oakland, California." From that day on, Jack has lived the health life and teaches Health & Fitness to millions every morning with his T.V. Exercise Show.

7

At its free end, the hair tapers to a fine needle point. At the bottom of the follicle or hair sheath in the scalp, the hair swells into a bulb or bowl which fits over the papilla—a bump or projection in one of the layers of the skin. This bulb is often erroneously called the root of the hair. Through the papilla the hair gets its nourishment from the blood.

When a hair comes out so that the bulb is visible, it has not "come out by the root." The bulb and papilla have merely parted company. So long as they are connected and the papilla is providing nourishment, the hair "lives." Separated from the papilla, it "dies" ... but if the papilla and follicle are functioning, another hair will take its place.

Connected with the follicles are muscles called arrectores pilorum, which make the expression "His hair stood on end" no idle figure of speech. The same muscles have another unpopular function—by contracting, they cause goose flesh.

There are three main varieties of hair: 1) Long, soft hair such as that of the head and beard, the pubes and the armpits; 2) Short, stiff hair as on the eyebrows and eyelashes; 3) Lanugo, the downy colorless hair found scattered over the body where other varieties are lacking. Hair is missing only from the palms, the soles and the eyelids of the normal body.

IMPORTANT FACTS ABOUT THE HAIR

A square inch of the average scalp holds about 1000 hairs, so that over the entire scalp there are some 120,000. Blondes have more hairs—sometimes as many as 140,000—and redheads only about 90,000. Black and brown heads run nearer the average. Flaxen hair is the finest, from 1/1500 to 1/500 of an inch in diameter ... and black hair is the coarsest, from 1/450 to 1/140 of an inch.

Hair is much more elastic than is usually realized. A hair can be stretched one-fifth of its length. It can support two to five ounces of weight without breaking.

As is generally known, the dampness or dryness of the atmosphere affects the curliness of the hair, since it is very sensitive to moisture. This characteristic has been put to use in the manufacture of hygrometers, instruments which measure the amount of moisture in the air.

That the friction between a comb and the hair produces static electricity is also well known. The static often gives off a crackling sound and frequently makes sparks in the dark.

Although various styles of hair dressing often seem highly artificial, there is evidence that they were originally influenced by the natural tendencies of the hair to grow in certain directions in certain places. There is a natural parting of the hair of the head. A part on the left side is found most commonly; one in the middle comes next; least common is a part on the right side. While it has never been any hairdresser's or beautician's inspiration to start a vogue of parting the eyebrows, the fact is that the hair of the left eyebrow shows as strong a tendency to part as does the hair on the left scalp. One hesitates to mention this characteristic lest Beauty Parlors begin to advertise eyebrow parting!

HAIR HAS PERIODS OF REST AND GROWTH

Hair growth, it might be said, is a series of reincarnations. Each normal hair, if untouched by disease or abuse, lives its full life span then drops out and is forgotten and replaced, like a human generation. The normal length of a hair's life however, has never been determined. It can vary from several months to four years. It has been calculated that the life of an eyelash is 150 days.

During the life of a hair, whatever the span, there are alternate periods of rest and growth. The periods of rest vary in different parts of the body, although there is a normal cycle for each.

The active period of growth seems to be about eight weeks. After that, if the hair is growing on the leg, for example, it rests for as long as three months. If it is a hair of the scalp, however, its rest period may be shorter or almost absent.

There may be several of these periods of growth and rest before the hair reaches its full length and is ready to drop out. Then, if a rest period arrives in time and the hair is not combed or pulled out, it may cling to the skin until the new hair pushes it out. The follicle has a tendency to contract about the old hair and help to hold it in. If a hair is pulled out or expelled, however, 41 to 72 days must elapse before the new hair emerges. This is at the usual rate of hair growth, which is 3/8 to 3/4 of an inch in a month. Hair grows faster by day than by night, and faster in the warmer summer months, it is said, and the rate of growth of a new hair is twice as fast as it is near the end of the hair's life.

Hair begins to grow long before birth. That is, the germs of the future hairs appear on the forehead and eyebrows in the tenth to twelfth week of the human embryo. Two weeks later the germs show above the lips, and in the sixteenth week on the rest of the head. After that the trunk, limbs and backs of the hands and feet show the hair germs. These are merely short, peg-like protuberances on the outer skin of the embryo.

Active growth of hair on the scalp begins immediately after it appears. The beard begins to appear at puberty, as does the hair of the genitals and the armpits.

HAIR DOES NOT GROW AFTER DEATH

We often hear of dead bodies which show a new growth of hair on the scalp or face. Don't you believe it! The idea that hair grows after death is a mistaken notion. What really happens in such cases is that the shrinking of the tissues after death makes the hairs, already in the skin, project farther. The color of the hair may change after death, however.

HEREDITY AND HAIR

Some very interesting facts as to the inheritance of types of hair have been reported by investigators who sent out thousands of questionnaires, collated the answers and checked the results by scientific investigation. They found, for example, that two blue eyed parents with straight, light hair will have only children of the same type. Two wavy haired parents may have children with straight, wavy or curly hair, but the chances are slight that there will be curly haired offspring. With two curly haired parents the proportion of curly heads will be larger, but they may also have children with wavy or even straight hair. If one parent has straight hair and the other curly, the children will all have curly hair if the curly haired parent is true to type—that is, himself the child of curly haired parents. Otherwise, some of the children will have straight hair, the rest curly.

As with individual strains, so with races and with mankind itself. What is normal by inheritance for one individual or race, or even sex, is abnormal for another. A beard means one thing on a man, another on a woman. Caucasians are normally heavily bearded; American Indians almost never. Lack of hair has run true down the centuries. The Chinese, the Mongols and the American Indians are the least hairy people both in the past and the present. The Indian is rarely bald. Negroes are more often bald than Indians. The hereditary tendencies may differ in degree, but not in kind. Some Negroes, for example, may have kinkier hair and some Indians coarser hair than others, but each inherits his kind.

This inheritance factor holds true throughout the animal kingdom. The Airedale, for example, has a distinctive coat well suited to the cold, damp climate in which the breed originated. Other breeds have different coats—short, long, straight, curly—a matter of environment and selection, with each member of the breed inheriting its kind of coat.

WHAT CIVILIZATION HAS DONE TO OUR HAIR

When we see human hair as it is today, it is hard to imagine it as it was in ancient times when it served man as it does animals—as clothing and armor and tentacles of the sense of touch. If you want to see what hair can be, examine the hair of a good Airedale dog—a soft, woolly undercoat, protecting against heat and cold, and a hard, wiry outer coat that sheds water like a rubber hat—altogether, almost like a suit of padded armor.

If the human race of today were compared to their ancient predecessors, it would be seen what part another basic factor —environment—has to do with the matter. From a hair's point of view, civilization has meant less and less exposure to life-giving sun rays and fresh air. Clothes and hats have taken the place of hair as insulation against heat and cold and moisture, and as a shield. The usefulness of hair is obviously not so great now as in earlier days, when artificial warmth was less common and blows on the skull more so.

Tight fitting hats have a habit of compressing the scalp, rubbing and wearing out hairs and choking the blood supply. False hair has added weight and warmth, and interferes with circulation, as well as being a frequent carrier of various infections. Although false hair happily went out of style some years ago when bobbing came popular, it is now back again and it is much in the mode today for women to wear wigs. Some women even have a "wig wardrobe" to go with the different styles and colors of their clothes wardrobe. A wig may be becoming—but it will do hair and scalp no more good than did the old fashioned rats, switches and transformations.

NOTIONS AND LOTIONS

Many factors, to be sure, affect the growth of normal hair— but a great many that are stressed by rumor and advertising simply have nothing to do with it.

One question on which dermatologists do not all agree is whether cutting stimulates growth of hair. Undoubtedly it has some effect. Some experimenters have proved to their satisfaction that cutting or shaving brings up hair faster, but others cannot find such evidence. Most young men who want more than "down" on their faces try shaving to produce a beard. Very likely their beards do grow a bit faster—but that would happen anyhow with increasing years, a fact that the young men seem to ignore.

Hairs do grow thicker and stiffer from shaving, however, and so does the hair of women who have their hair bobbed or other fashionable short haircuts. When so-called superfluous hair is temporarily removed by shaving, pulling or chemical depilatories, the succeeding hairs are also thicker and stiffer.

Some barbers and beauticians are ingenious in devising novel forms of personal attention—such as mud packs, eyelash baths, ear rubs, nose pulls and what not—and often advise their patrons that cut hair should be singed in order to close the pores and retain the vitality of the hair. All this would be highly scientific and helpful if hairs had pores, or could exude vitality. But it so happens that the hair is a solid mass of cells and has no tube or duct through which to lose the vitality which it does not possess.

Equally incorrect are the advertisers of various lotions and tonics who assert that their preparations make hair grow. *There is no chemical which, directly applied, will make a new hair.* Neither will tonics or any so-called secret hair preparation, no matter how skillfully convincing the advertising may be. Vigorous rubbing with any sort of mild concoction as a lubricant may possibly help stimulate slow growth by increasing the blood supply, but it is probably the rubbing more than the chemical that is responsible.

There is some relation between the oily secretion of the sweat glands and hair growth, however. People with excessive hair growth often show heavy sweating. Heat has a stimulating effect on hair, so that it grows slightly faster in summer than in winter. Cold acts as a tonic when it improves the circulation of the scalp.

HEALTHY HAIR BEGINS WITH A CLEAN BLOOD STREAM

This book will have accomplished a great deal if it can drive home just this one point:

Healthy Hair Needs A Healthy Constitution

How does the constitution influence the well being of the hair? Briefly, the hair—like a bud or branch—depends for its health on the trunk or limb from which it grows. That trunk or limb, in the case of the hair, is the skin—an organ, a member of the body. The nourishment on which the hair lives is supplied by the body through the skin—the blood and oxygen carried by the blood vessels in the papilla to the cells from which the hair grows. Clearly, anything which affects —the quality and quantity of the blood affects the hair growth. And the chief factor in the production of good, nourishing blood is Health!

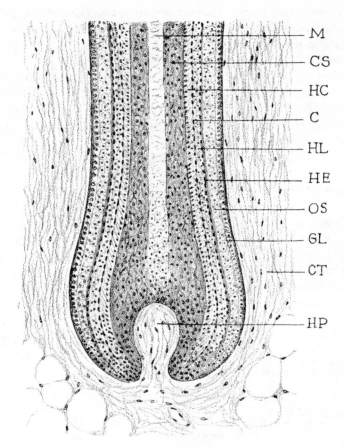

M

CS

HC

C

HL

HE

OS

GL

CT

HP

SECTION THROUGH LOWER PART OF FOLLICLE

M—Medulla

CS—Cortical substance

HC—Hair cuticle

C—Cuticle of the follicle

HL—Layer of Huxley

HE—Layer of Henle

OS—Outer sheath

GL—Glassy membrane

CT—Connective tissue

HP—Hair papilla

Patricia and I have done a tremendous amount of research on the human hair and scalp ... research which has taken us throughout the civilized world, and among primitive peoples as well.

We have found that the people who live their whole lives bareheaded in the sunlight and eat an abundance of natural foods—that is, a natural balanced diet—seldom, if ever, suffer from baldness, thin hair, dandruff or other problems of the hair and scalp.

"HAIR SOIL" DOES NOT MEAN DIRT!

Sometimes a person's general health is good, yet the hairline is receding. Why does this happen? Bad habits, such as very little brushing, are usually responsible. Dirty, unwashed hair invites parasites to begin colonizing and raising families on that head!

You parents of children with long hair must protect their valuable crop by seeing to it that their hair is washed and brushed regularly. And should it be a boy—that is a very good and logical health reason to tell him to get a proper boy's short haircut.

I STARTED LOSING MY HAIR WHEN I WAS 16

At the age of sixteen I was suffering from tuberculosis. With this degenerating condition that was destroying my body, I noticed that my hair was dull and lifeless. I was sick, and it was reflected in my hair. As previously stated, the hair is a good mirror for the condition of one's health.

When I combed and brushed my hair, large amounts of it came out. Now, I want you to understand that it is perfectly natural to lose some dead hair from your head every day of your life. This will be explained more fully in the book when we outline a Program of Hair Care. But there is a limit to the amount of hair that should come out each day.

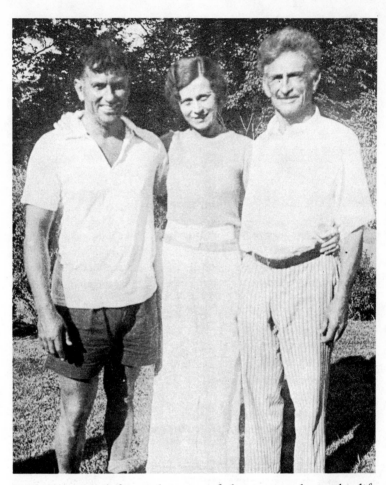

Paul C. Bragg (left) at the turn of the century began his lifetime career in Natural Physical Fitness with the famous Physical Culture pioneer, Bernarr Macfadden (right). Bragg was editor of Macfadden's Physical Culture Magazine, which was the first publication to bring to popular attention and interest the basic principles of healthful living in the U.S.A. He is credited with "getting women out of bloomers into shorts, and men into bathing trunks." Bragg was also active with Macfadden's "Penny Kitchen Restaurants" during the Depression era, when they fed millions of hungry people. He worked with Macfadden in America's first Health Spa at Dansville, N.Y., where the above photo was taken.

I rushed to the barber shop hoping to get some help. Then I became a slave to hair tonics. If a tonic was new, I bought it on sight. I tried every kind of shampoo that I heard of. I was a victim of the barber's wiles. The money my parents spent trying to save my hair—all to no purpose! My hair continued to come out just as fast as it did before I tried all these "remedies." Every time I combed my hair it told the same story—my body was sick and my hair was not getting the proper nourishment.

HOW MY HAIR WAS SAVED

When I arrived at Dr. August Rollier's great Natural Healing Sanatorium in Leysen, Switzerland, I confided to the doctor that I was worried and distressed not only about the condition of my general health, but also about the tragedy of my loss of hair. I feared that if it continued I would be bald. Think of it . . . going bald before the age of twenty!

And yet today, as I look at the boys and young men of this generation, I see the same thing happening to their hair as was happening to mine then. I am a great lover of sports and during the last few months I have attended athletic events where there were large numbers of High School and young College men. I was shocked to see how many of them were losing their hair. Some were receding at the front part of the head, others showing thin spots on the crown of the scalp. It would not be long before they would have large bald spots. I noticed how lifeless was the hair of these boys.

And the young girls were having many hair problems. So many had their hair cut short, and on close examination I could see how thin their crop of hair was. Again I saw receding hair at the front of the head.

Among these thousands of young men and women I saw only a few with beautiful hair and plenty of it.

Then I saw them eat the hot dog sandwiches, the cola drinks, the ice cream, the candy bars and all the other devitalized foods.

Here were boys and girls in this day and age having hair and scalp problems the same as I in the long time ago.

Dr. Rollier was sympathetic toward me and my hair problem. He said he was amazed to learn how little really authoritative information was known about the proper care of the hair and scalp. He told me that one need not let the hair grow thin or the scalp suffer from many problems. He informed me that if the hair is falling out and you are having scalp problems, a reasonable amount of proper care will restore it, unless one is completely bald.

And the same care will keep the hair strong and healthy throughout life. He spoke of simple, natural methods for treating the hair and scalp by following a few Laws of Nature.

I followed Dr. Rollier's advice to the letter, and today—having lived threescore and ten years plus—I have a thick, luxuriant head of healthy hair.

And the same goes for my daughter Patricia, who is co-author of this book. She has beautiful luxuriant hair.

- We both follow the hair program that we lay before you in this book.

- We both are constantly seeking new methods to aid in improving the health of your hair and scalp.

- We feel that we can help YOU to help yourself have a healthy head of hair, and that you can have hair that is wonderfully silky in texture, and that your scalp can be cleansed of every trace of dandruff and roughness.

TOXIC POISON—THE GREATEST ENEMY OF HAIR

I spoke of attending athletic events where there were large crowds of young men and women, who consumed great amounts of hot dogs, cremated hamburgers, ice cream, cola drinks, soft drinks, candy and other devitalized foods.

Little do these young people realize that they are filling their blood streams with toxic poisons that will help destroy, not only their exuberant health, but also their hair.

Give some weeds an inch, and they will take a yard.

HOW DEVITALIZED FOODS DESTROYED THE HAIR OF A BROTHER AND SISTER

At our family home in Hollywood, California, we have many fine neighbors. Near our home lived a very famous film director with his wife and two children, a boy and a girl. We saw these children grow from childhood to adults, and had an opportunity to see the tragic effect of a nutritionally deficient diet on the hair.

When these children were very young they had the most beautiful heads of hair. Their mother was health conscious and fed her children correctly—and it showed not only in their exceptionally good health, but also in their very good-looking, strong, healthy hair. They had the thickest and most luxuriant hair ever seen on children's heads. People would stop to exclaim how beautiful their hair was.

Their hair remained in this beautiful condition until this brother and sister entered High School. There, someway, somehow, the parents seemed to lose control of feeding their children. They had never had devitalized foods at home. But when they mixed with other High School boys and girls, they grew rebellious and completely went off their healthful natural diet. They followed the masses ... and soon were eating hot dogs, drinking cola drinks and gorging on all the other foodless foods that teenagers consume these days.

Very soon there was a change in their hair. It was no longer a thing of beauty. Why? Several things were happening in their blood streams. These foodless foods left a large amount of uneliminated toxic poisons in the blood stream. As the blood coursed throughout the circulatory system, these toxic poisons were deposited in the "hair soil" of the scalp. These toxic poisons did not nourish the hair.

The degeneration of the hair of these young people was a long, slow process. First, the hair seemed to lose its sheen and lustre. It grew coarse and straw-like. When they graduated from High School and entered College, they continued their bad eating habits and even added smoking to their bad habits of living.

In their last year of College there was a pronounced change

19

in their hair. The boy's hair was not only receding, but a bald spot had appeared on the crown of his scalp. Gone was the thick, strong hair of his pre-High School days. He was going bald rapidly. His sister's hair was now cut short. It was dead and lifeless ... no longer her "Crowning Glory" as hair should be to every woman. It was unmanageable. As she cut it shorter and shorter, you could see the damage that was being done by bad diet, malnutrition, mineral, vitamin and protein deficiencies.

Today the young man is a businessman and is completely bald. His sister is a housewife and her hair beauty is entirely gone. She wears a wig most of the time when she goes out.

I could tell you about many sad cases exactly like this. It is the same with pets, dogs and cats. You can tell how these animals are being fed by looking at their fur. If it has a sheen that sparkles, those animals are being fed correctly and are free from toxic poisons.

Patricia and I are members of many fine clubs in Southern California, and we see the tragedy of people who have every means to take care of themselves, but are letting toxic poisons ruin their hair, scalp and general health.

(See back cover of this book for information about *The Bragg Toxicless Diet Body Purification and Healing System* booklet which will help you to learn more about how to avoid body degeneration.)

AVOID THESE FOODS IF YOU WANT STRONG, HEALTHY HAIR

REFINED SUGAR is one of the most deficient and toxic foods on the face of the earth. It leaches the calcium from your hair, blood, bones and teeth. Regard it as you would a poison. Keep it out of your diet!

REFINED FLOUR is the second great toxic and deficient food. Have no part of it in any shape or form! Nature never grew a white grain of wheat. Man in his ignorance and commercial greed *bled it white*.

HYDROGENATED OR HIGH POINT OILS. Read labels on all foods. The law requires that if the oil is hydrogenated and passed in interstate commerce, it must so state on the label. Your body has a heat of 98.6 degrees. For your body to utilize hydrogenated oils, you would have to have a body heat of 300 degrees. Therefore, you must see how impossible it is for your body to assimilate hydrogenated oils. Your hair and scalp need natural oil for nourishment. The oils that help nourish the hair and scalp are the natural cold pressed oils such as olive oil, sesame oil, soya oil, safflower oil, corn oil, peanut oil, sunflower seed oil and walnut oil.

SALT. Common table salt is an enemy of strong, healthy hair. In our intensive research on healthy hair, we find that people who use excessive amounts of salt have scalp troubles and are inclined to lose their hair. Salt has a drying effect on the entire body and dries out the hair and scalp.

HAM, BACON, HOT DOGS, CORNED BEEF AND LUNCH MEATS. All these food products are heavily fortified with salt, brine and concentrated salt chemicals to preserve them. SODIUM NITRATE and SODIUM NITRITE are used in practically all prepared cured lunch meats.

WHITE RICE. Here is another toxic food. The important B Complex Vitamins have been removed from the outer part of the rice. Your hair needs the B Complex Vitamins.

ALCOHOLIC BEVERAGES, COLA DRINKS, SOFT DRINKS, TEA, COFFEE AND CHOCOLATE. None of these beverages can add any nourishment to your hair and scalp. They are heavily laden with toxic materials that may easily do damage to your hair and scalp.

KEEP AWAY FROM MANUFACTURED FOODS. The grocery and supermarket shelves are filled with processed foods such as prepared cereals, prepared desserts, degerminated cereals. Practically all the cornmeal found on the standard grocery shelf has been degerminated. All this processing is done to give these so-called foods a long shelf life. They have been *robbed of their* VITAL LIFE. They are stomach fillers but not body nourishers. To grow strong, thick, healthy hair you need foods which contain all the natural nourishment that Nature puts into natural foods. There are over 700 chemicals or food additives used today by the food processors.

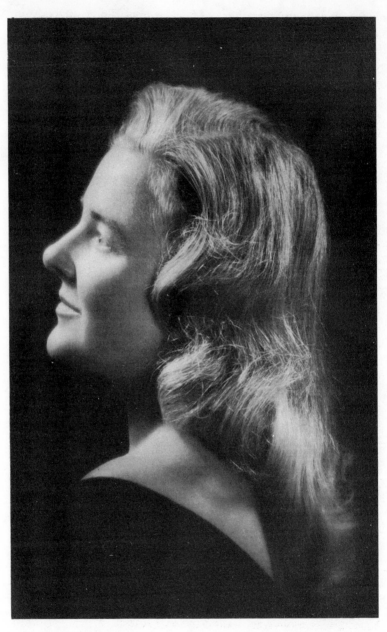

Patricia Bragg has long, thick, healthy, luxuriant hair.

SULPHUR DIOXIDE is an inorganic chemical used extensively in preserving dried fruits.

BENZOATE OF SODA is a chemical used to preserve hundreds of different kinds of foods found on the shelves of the supermarket. It is extensively used in butter substitutes.

HARDENED FAT FOODS. Practically all butter substitutes are made from HYDROGENATED OR HIGH POINT OILS. It is better nutritionally to use the unsaturated oils and salt free butter.

EATING TO BUILD A HEALTHY HEAD OF HAIR AND SCALP

To have a head of strong, healthy hair and a clean, healthy scalp, follow Nature's Laws of Natural Eating. Avoid as you would the plague such unnatural foods as cured meats, sausage, etc ... tea, coffee, cocoa, whiskey, beer, wines, cola and soft drinks ... such denatured and degerminated foods as white bread and white rice ... all devitalized, processed foodless foods ... also vegetables and meats that have had the life cooked out of them, especially when their natural juices have been removed.

DON'T EAT FRIED FOODS. The frying pan is the cradle of indigestion, heart disease and death. The sputtering lumps of frying, sizzling fat are enemies of your hair, scalp and entire body.

SALT acts like a sponge, absorbing water from the blood and setting up an insatiable desire for liquid. Insatiable because, even when the system holds all the water possible, the unsettled salt-induced craving persists. Fried foods add to the trouble. All these unnatural conditions help destroy the health and beauty of your hair and scalp.

KEEP YOUR FOODS AS NATURAL AS POSSIBLE

Educate your taste buds to distinguish the delicate flavors of natural foods. Those foods which have to be doused with catsup, mustard and hot sauces are usually processed foods that are not fit to eat. The cleaner you get your 260 taste buds, the more natural your diet will become. In time you will develop a natural instinct for the correct selection of food. It will become impossible for you to swallow anything except the clean, wholesome, nourishing foods that Nature has provided.

YOUR HAIR IS MADE FROM THE FOOD YOU EAT

Remember that your hair and your scalp are made from the food that you eat. We professionals in the field of Nutrition use the expression, *"You are what you eat."* If you want a full head of thick, strong, goodlooking hair you will eat only those natural, nourishing foods that will supply your hair and scalp with essential nutrients.

FEED THE HAIR AND SCALP TOXICLESS FOODS

As explained earlier in this book, you have a "hair soil" which lies underneath your scalp. Just like the soil of Mother Earth, this hair soil must be fed the essential nutrients so it will grow healthy, thick, strong hair. If you feed the soil of the hair and scalp on toxic foods it is going to show up in the condition of the hair and scalp. If you eat toxic forming foods you cannot expect to have thick, strong, healthy hair and a healthy scalp.

Also, when the body's vitality is lowered it shows up in the hair and scalp. If toxic poisons are brought into the hair soil and hair structure by way of the blood, the hair structure is more than likely to suffer because the scalp is unable to resist and throw off these toxins. The hair and scalp of a person with a weak constitution are in exactly the same difficulty as that person would be if he were fed poison in his food, for blood is the food supply of the scalp and hair.

When the hair falls out during and after such conditions as influenza, it is because the weakened system has been unable to defend the hair against the attacks of toxins. When anemia, heart, lung or kidney conditions have enfeebled the constitution, it is quite common for the hair to fall out or to change its appearance and quality. In fact, any disturbance in the metabolism—the mechanism controlling the building up and breaking down of the body—usually results in some alteration of the hair. Particularly noteworthy are the changes that occur in the hair when the function of the glands of internal secretion is disarranged.

Poor blood makes poor hair, just as poor food makes poor bodies. Many cases of dry, lusterless hair which falls out easily are due to nutritional deficiencies.

PROTEIN—THE HAIR BUILDER

Protein is the material you are made of. Protein is the Number One Diet Item for a thick, healthy head of hair. Protein means "to come first"—and if it doesn't, you are in for all kinds of problems of the hair and scalp.

Every part of your body relies on protein for proper growth and normal functioning. You must eat adequate amounts of either animal or vegetable proteins if you are to have a head of thick, healthy hair.

Protein is found in liver, heart, sweetbreads, beef, lamb, poultry, fish, eggs, cheese, nuts, seeds, brewer's yeast, wheat germ, brown rice, peanut butter, soybeans, cornmeal, whole wheat, avocados and buckwheat flour. In fact, all foods contain some protein. Those listed here are the highest in protein content.

It has been found that the races who get adequate amounts of protein in their daily diet usually have healthy hair and plenty of it all the days of their lives. On the other hand, people who eat large amounts of carbohydrates (starches and sugars) in their regular diet do not have such healthy hair as do the protein eaters.

A TRUE STORY OF TWINS AND WHAT
HAPPENED TO THEIR HAIR

Many years ago I had twin brothers in my employ. When they came to work for me both had thick, healthy hair with a glossy sheen. I will call these boys Bill and Joe. Their hair tells the story of their lives—a quite different story for each, although they were twins and started off with basically the same natural physical attributes.

Bill was the more intelligent of the twins, and became intensely interested in my nutritional work and health culture. I told Bill that God had blessed him with unusually healthy, thick hair—but in order to keep it perfect, he would have to know how to feed and keep the hair healthy.

I explained that the minimum daily Protein Ration for a man is 64 grams and for a woman 55 grams. (There are 28 grams to the ounce.) I told Bill that he could eat up to 150 grams per day—and that Nutritional Science considers the animal proteins most active biologically, but that vegetable proteins are also complete proteins. He could make his own personal choice of proteins—either animal or vegetable or both.

I pointed out that he must learn to live on a balanced diet.

WHAT IS A BALANCED DIET?

In the present state of our knowledge we can say with the greatest assurance that a complete and balanced diet is one that shall satisfy the following specifications:

1. It must furnish enough energy to keep the body going.
2. It must furnish material for growth and for replacement of tissue waste.
3. It must furnish enough water.
4. It must furnish enough minerals.
5. It must furnish all the important vitamins.
6. It must furnish enough bulk, moisture and lubrication for normal elimination of the bowels.
7. It must contain all the important nutrients so that the scalp is healthy and the hair is thick and strong with a glossy, healthy sheen.

By now you know that there is only one way to have good health, as well as a healthy scalp and a head of thick, healthy hair. And that is by providing each of the billions of cells in your body with all the necessary nutrients.

---

*Life is like a gun. It can be aimed in only one direction
at a time. Make your aim—health!*

Remember, hair is built by the food you eat. Learn to use the natural live foods that contain the highest and best food values.

Remember, the *Number One Food for Healthy Hair is PROTEIN.* Your best sources of PROTEIN are: beef, lamb, poultry, fish, liver, heart, kidneys, sweetbreads, eggs, dairy products, brewer's yeast, avocado, peanuts and peanut butter, soybeans, cornmeal, seeds and nuts of all kinds, wheat germ, legumes (beans of all kinds) and brown rice.

THE NEXT MOST IMPORTANT NUTRIENT FOR HEALTHY HAIR—ORGANIC SULPHUR

Like Protein, ORGANIC SULPHUR is an important part of the hair. Organic Sulphur—(as distinguished from the inorganic chemical—Sulphur Dioxide which is harmful)—acts as a blood cleanser or conditioner. It helps promote the secretion of bile and is an aid to the liver in absorbing minerals.

Nutritionists call Organic Sulphur the Beauty Mineral because it is vitally necessary for strong, healthy, thick hair. It is also necessary for a good, clear, clean, youthful looking complexion and stronger fingernails.

A good source of this natural Organic Sulphur is in animal and vegetable proteins. It is found in egg yolk, cauliflower, cabbage, turnips, brussels sprouts, onions and garlic.

OTHER ESSENTIALS FOR HAIR HEALTH— CALCIUM, NATURAL FATS, SILICON

CALCIUM is found in all natural cheese, milk (certified raw is best), green leafy vegetables (such as mustard greens, turnip greens and kale), soybeans and molasses. Its proper absorption in the body depends greatly on Vitamin D, which is also contained in some of these foods.

CALCIUM is essential for healthy nerves and strong fingernails, as well as healthy hair. It is required more than any other mineral for the repair of body tissues. We need about 4 grams of Calcium in our daily diet in order to maintain general good health—and the health of your hair and scalp depend upon the health of your body.

NATURAL FATS are also needed in the body chemistry for healthy hair. Natural vegetable oils are the best source—such as safflower oil, soya oil, peanut oil, sesame oil, corn oil, olive oil—along with seeds and nuts of all kinds, avocado, fish liver oil and wheat germ oil. Natural animal fats—such as butter, cream, egg yolk, fat fish and fat meats—should be limited after age forty.

A limited amount of CARBOHYDRATES (starches and sugars) are required for healthy hair. These are found chiefly in natural whole grains of all kinds, dry legumes (beans of all kinds), vegetables, brown rice and fruits.

SILICON is a highly important organic mineral for growing a head of thick, glossy, healthy hair. In body chemistry, Silicon helps to build hair, nails, skin and teeth, and makes tissues supple. It aids grace, litheness, keen hearing and sparkling eyes, hard teeth and strong, thick, glossy hair.

FOODS HIGH IN SILICON: Green leaf vegetables top this list. Your daily diet should always include a large green leafy combination salad, composed of green lettuce, raw spinach leaves, parsley, watercress, green celery, green onions, green sweet bell peppers and any other green leafy raw vegetables.

Whole natural Barley is also an excellent source of Silicon, for animals as well as humans. Whole natural Barley can be purchased at all fine Health Food Stores. (Do not use pearled Barley, because the outer skin has been removed and that is where most of the Silicon is stored.)

Whole Brown Rice is rich in Silicon, and so are steel cut natural oats, millet, whole rye, whole corn, whole wheat and Fruits, especially grapes. Goat's milk is high in Silicon; next comes cow's raw milk, then pastuerized milk.

The less we leave to chance, the more certain success will be.

IODINE IS A NECESSITY FOR HEALTHY HAIR

IODINE is an important organic mineral for producing thick, strong hair with a sparkling sheen. In fact, Iodine is one of the essential organic minerals of the human body— necessary to resist germs and to render harmless the toxins they produce ... necessary for effective metabolism ... necessary to digestion and assimilation ... and necessary for efficient mental development.

An *Iodine deficiency* in an adult may be determined by simple symptomatic conditions before it reaches serious proportions. These include that "chronic tired feeling" ... the lack of usual ambition, pep, energy, with little refreshment from rest ... getting up in the morning more tired than when going to bed. In some people, there can be an accumulation of SOFT, FLABBY FLESH ... FALLING HAIR ... PREMATURE GRAYING OF THE HAIR ... BRITTLE, HARD-TO-MANAGE HAIR ... AND HAIR THAT SEEMS TO HAVE LOST ALL ITS LIFE.

Most people have the impression that Iodine is merely a chemical which in some mysterious way prevents goiter, and it is officially reported that there are 40 million people in the United States today who suffer from simple goiter. True, Iodine is essential in prevention of goiter. But, as noted above, it is also necessary in many other ways. Today we know that the presence in the diet of a slight trace of this important mineral can make the difference between a highly intelligent person and a drooling idiot.

The average body contains about 25 milligrams of Iodine (0.00004 percent of the total body weight). Two-thirds of it (15 milligrams) is concentrated in the thyroid gland. The other third is distributed in the tissues and blood.

We know that you are interested in this organic mineral so that you will have healthy, thick, glossy hair. So let us examine WHERE WE CAN GET IODINE IN OUR DAILY FOOD.

Thought and learning are small value unless translated into action.
—Wang Ming, Chinese philosopher

ALL OCEAN FOODS, both animal and vegetables, are rich in Iodine. Seaweed has 21,800 micrograms of Iodine to the pound. So seaweed can be our best source of Iodine, and many kinds are for sale on the market today. Nova Scotia Dulse may be purchased at Health Food Stores in the whole leaf or powdered. Pacific Ocean Kelp is the most popular way of getting your daily ration of Iodine, because it comes powdered in a shaker top box and can be sprinkled over your food. The simplest form, of course, to take natural organic Iodine is in small tablet form. Every Health Food Store features these Iodine Kelp tablets. A 5-grain tablet is recommended.

As noted, all seafoods contain organic Iodine. Whenever possible, try to obtain fresh fish.

PROTEIN, CALCIUM, NATURAL FATS, ORGANIC SULPHUR, SILICON AND IODINE ARE THE FOODS FOR YOUR HAIR AND SCALP—SO GET THEM IN YOUR DAILY DIET.

In the case of preserving the hair, an ounce of prevention is worth a ton of cure. Remember, each hair is supported by the blood stream. And the blood stream must have the essential nutrients to feed each hair correctly.

HERE IS THE BALANCED DIET I PLANNED FOR BILL FROM THESE FOODS

This SEVEN DAY MENU—given on the following pages —is what I explained to Bill was a Balanced Natural Diet to help in keeping his vitality high, his health perfect, and retaining the wonderful head of beautiful hair that God had blessed him with. This is the menu which I would suggest for anyone who is interested in GOOD HEALTH, VITALITY and HAVING HEALTHY HAIR.

There are no more important ingredients of a properly constituted diet than fruits and vegetables, for they contain vitamins of every class, recognized and unrecognized.—Sir Robert McCarrison

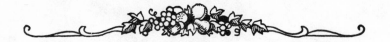

1st DAY

Breakfast

Natural Sun-Dried Apricots*
topped with Raw Wheat Germ and
Sliced Banana or Orange (if desired)
(If still hungry, add)
1 Egg and 1 Slice of Whole Grain Toast

*Soaked overnight in distilled water.

Lunch

Raw Vegetable Combination Salad
consisting of
Watercress, Grated Raw Beet, Grated Carrot,
Tomato and Green Onions

Salad Dressing
made of
Fresh Lemon and Oil with a trace of Honey

½ Cup of Sunflower Seeds
(rich in Protein and Natural Oil)

Raw Apple

Dinner

Tossed Green-Leaf Salad
with
Raw Chopped Spinach, Lettuce, Cucumber,
Celery, Tomato

Lemon and Oil Dressing

Protein—Either Animal or Vegetable

Fresh Fruit

You are what you eat! What you eat today will be walking and talking tomorrow.

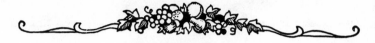

2nd DAY

Breakfast

Apple Sauce with Honey*

Steel Cut Oats**
with
Natural Molasses

Whole Wheat Toast

* Make your own Apple Sauce and add Honey as used.
**Top with Sliced Banana or other Fruit, if desired.

Lunch

Raw Vegetable Combination Salad
(Same as 1st Day)

Vegetable Soup with plenty of Natural Barley

Whole Rye Toast

Dinner

Cabbage Cole Slaw with Onions

Baked Fish
with
Lemon and Herbs

Stewed Tomatoes   Cauliflower

Fresh Fruit

(*or*)

Avocado and Tomato Salad

Asparagus   Broccoli

Nuts of any kind

Fresh Fruit

Thy food shall be thy remedy.—Hippocrates

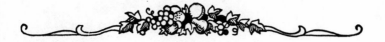

3rd DAY

Breakfast

Natural Black Mission Figs

Broiled Liver (Medium Rare)
or
Sunflower Seeds

Raw Apple

Lunch

Raw Vegetable Combination Salad
(Same as 1st Day)

1 Hard Boiled Egg
or
Nut Butter

Whole Grain Toast

Dinner

Tossed Green-Leaf Salad
(Same as 1st Day)

Broiled Lean Meat (Medium Rare)
or
Mixed Nuts

Green Beans   Steamed Beets

Grapes
or any Fruit in season

---

*If your food is devitalized, the important elements of nourishment have
been removed, or if its value has been diminished by wrong
cooking processes—you can then starve to death on a full stomach.*

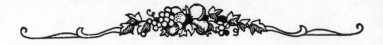

4th DAY

Breakfast

Stewed Prunes
topped with
Sliced Bananas
Raw Wheat Germ and Honey

Natural Cheese
(not processed)

Sunflower Seeds

Lunch

Lettuce, Tomato and Cucumber Salad

Lemon and Oil Dressing

Baked Onions (Keep Whole)

Lamb Chop
or
Mixed Nuts or Seeds

Baked Apple*

*Stuff center with Raisins, top with Honey after baking.

Dinner

Raw Vegetable Combination Salad
(Same as 1st Day)

Natural Brown Rice

Baked Eggplant**

Fresh Fruit and Dates

**Slice Eggplant in half before putting in oven to bake. For last 10 minutes, top with chopped tomatoes. Eat skin and all!

---

*Don't injure your system by over-feeding it. Over-eating
will kill you long before your time.*

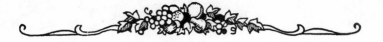

5th DAY

Breakfast

Raw Apple

Whole Grain Cereal
topped with
Sliced Banana and Honey

Lunch

Cabbage Cole Slaw
with
Grated Carrots and Apple

Lentils and Brown Rice
(cooked together)
or
Broiled Liver (Medium Rare) with Onions

Dinner

Green-Leaf Combination Salad
with Tomatoes

Baked Potato (Eat the skin)

Baked Brussels Sprouts

Corn Bread*

*Made with stone ground cornmeal—-not from degerminated cornmeal.

Habits of rapid eating are most harmful, and must be overcome.
Quietness and Cheerfulness at meals is most essential.
—Oliver Wendell Holmes

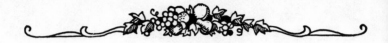

6th DAY

Breakfast

Natural Sun-Dried Apricots*
topped with Raw Wheat Germ
and sliced Banana or Orange

1 Egg

Whole Grain Toast

*Soak in water overnight. (Be sure they are sun-dried and free of preservatives.)

Lunch

Raw Vegetable Combination Salad
(Same as 1st Day)

Steamed Green Squash

Sunflower Seeds and Raisins

Dinner

Chopped Raw Spinach Salad
with other Raw Vegetables

Hamburger Patties (Medium Rare)
or
Mixed Nuts and Seeds

Kale

Steamed Yellow Squash

Fresh Fruit and Dates

Ninety per cent of our disorders are due to errors in diet. The majority eat more than is good for them—Sir Hy. Thompson, M.D.

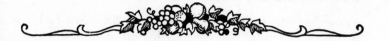

7th DAY

Breakfast

Grapes

1 Egg or Nuts

Whole Grain Toast

Lunch

Salad of Cabbage, Tomatoes
Celery and Green Bell Peppers

Tuna Fish Sandwich
or
Sunflower Seeds

Fresh Fruit and Dates

Dinner

Sliced Tomatoes

Roast Lamb
or
Mixed Nuts and Seeds

Steamed Green Peas and Sliced Carrots

Apple Sauce
(Sweeten with Honey)

WIDE VARIETY OF HEALTHFUL AND DELICIOUS RECIPES

The *Bragg Health Food Cook Book* contains 444 pages of information and healthful, delicious recipes for you to choose from—see back page of this book for details.

Some people require more food than others. Maybe a nice Combination Salad first, then your Protein Entree, ending up with an Apple is sufficient. Or you might want to add one or two Vegetables. The SEVEN DAY MENU given here offers a variety of basic combinations of healthful natural foods from which you may make your own balanced selection.

HEALTH DRINKS, BEVERAGES AND HERB TEAS

These have their place in a healthful diet. We feel that it is not wise to drink beverages with your main meals. But if during the day you wish a hot cup of herb tea or if you wish a glass of freshly squeezed orange or grapefruit juice, etc., that's fine, go ahead and enjoy it.

THE BRAGG FAVORITE JUICE COCKTAIL—consists of all raw vegetables which we prepare in our vegetable juicer: Carrots, Spinach, Watercress, Beets and Celery.

THE BRAGG FAVORITE HEALTH "PEP" DRINK—We often have it in the morning instead of breakfast, and it is a delicious beverage meal anytime.

Bragg Healthy Hair "Pep" Drink

Prepare in blender:

Juice of 2-3 Oranges (fresh) or unsweetened Pineapple Juice or Distilled Water	*1/3 tsp. pure Pectin Powder*
	1 teaspoon Whey
	1 Banana
1 Egg (fertile, if possible)	*1 teaspoon pure Vanilla*
3 tablespoons Raw Wheat Germ	*1 teaspoon Honey*
1 teaspoon Brewers Yeast	*1 tablespoon Soya Powder*
1 teaspoon Liquid Lecithin	*1 tablespoon Protein Powder*

Optional:

4 Apricots (sun dried, unsulphured). Soak overnight in distilled water. We soak enough to last for several days. Keep refrigerated in jar.

NOTE: In summer you can add fresh fruit—peaches, strawberries, berries, apricots or any other fresh fruit in season instead of the banana.

Each of us has a perfectly natural tendency to underestimate our own powers—to feel despair—to want to quit—but this is just when you should go on to success and satisfaction.

SUPERIOR NUTRITION—THE FOUNDATION OF
SUPERIOR HEALTH AND ACHIEVEMENT

In giving Bill this Seven Day Menu I tried to give him a wide variety of foods, so that he would get plenty of Protein, Calcium, Organic Sulphur, Natural Fats and Silicon along will all the foods necessary for a completely balanced diet.

Remember, when Bill came to me he was under twenty, and had absolutely no instruction in Nutrition. Not only did he follow my diet for physical health, but he also mentally devoured everything on Nutrition in my complete Health Library. As the years went by, the more he learned about Nutrition the more he applied this knowledge for the good of his own body.

Bill is a self-made man. Besides working part time for me, he completed a University course in Law and graduated with honors, passed his bar examination and went to work in a law office. He continued to follow my complete instructions on the care of the hair as given in this book.

Joe, too, was a fine young man. But unlike his brother Bill, Joe was not the least interested in Nutrition and Health Culture. He had graduated from High School and had no further interest in higher education. He took to smoking (although never in my presence, as I will not tolerate tobacco smoke where I can control it).

TIME MARCHES ON. It has been 35 years since these twins worked for me. Remember I told you that when they entered my employ, both had thick, beautiful hair.

Today Bill is an outstanding attorney. He is still a fine athlete and I often play tennis with him or go on long mountain hikes. He still has one of the most beautiful heads of hair of any man I know. And that's saying a lot, because my lecture work takes me all over the world and I meet thousands of men.

Bill maintains that wonderful head of hair, which is the envy of most men who meet him. People even stop him on the street to ask how he keeps such thick, healthy hair.

NOW LOOK AT JOE'S LIFE TODAY

Joe still eats the regular foodless foods of civilization. Even with two heart attacks, he still uses salty foods and smokes a few cigarettes daily.

Joe has not done very well with his life. He is in a dead-end job at a box factory. He has had two unsuccessful marriages, and is now on his third. One of his children by his first marriage died, and one is a victim of polio.

I'm sure you are anxious to know about Joe's hair. Well, there is very little to say—because Joe is completely bald. Yes, along about 27 he started losing his great head of healthy, strong hair.

You ask, "Did he feel badly about losing his hair?"

Oh, yes! His "Crowning Glory" was one of his most prized personal assets. He made a hard fight to save it. He used preparations of all kinds, went to hair specialists who put lights, creams and lotions on it, and used heavy massage—all to no avail. Joe was not feeding his hair. Soon it was all gone.

He felt so badly about his bald head that he purchased a toupee. But his fellow workers kept teasing him and asking, "Joe, who do you think you're fooling with that rug?" So, Joe discarded the toupee and now suffers in silence.

DON'T FOLLOW JOE'S EXAMPLE

I have seen this same tragedy occur time and time again ... among members of exclusive clubs ... professional men ... tradesmen ... factory workers ... all walks of life. Too many people think they can just brush their hair and shampoo it and it will stay thick and healthy. But it does not happen that way.

We have repeatedly told you in this book that to have healthy hair, you must feed it the nutrients that will make it grow healthy and thick.

It is our honest conviction that if all men and women would feed their bodies correctly and follow a Program of Hair Hygiene, it would be practically impossible to have unhealthy hair and scalp.

In our years of teaching Hair Culture we have seen some startling things happen to people who had sick hair. When they became alerted to the importance of Good Nutrition and a Program of Hair Culture, a miracle seemed to happen to their hair and scalp.

FOLLOW NATURE'S LAWS

It's just following Nature's Laws. We have no cures for baldness. Our system is one of prevention.

The proof that many people are suffering from malnutrition is evidenced by the fact that 80% of our population will, during a 12-month period, have one or more "colds," with 30% having influenza. And the mortality rate from infectious diseases is enormously high.

As we have stressed, the condition of your general health reflects in your hair and scalp. This is as true for humans as it is for animals. Many times in my life I have taken dogs and cats who were fed incorrectly and had miserable coats of fur, and by good nutrition, hygiene and proper care have made those ugly creatures into things of beauty.

Several years ago I went to the Los Angeles Pound and selected the sickest dog with the ugliest coat that I could find. Even the sympathetic attendants wanted to know why I wanted such a miserable creature when there were so many better looking and healthier dogs. I did not answer their questions at the time—but waited to let the dog show what could be done by good nutrition and hair hygiene. In six months I brought that dog back to the Pound—and the attendants would not believe that it was the same dog. But it was! The contrast was the result of correct nutrition and proper hair care. And we have done the same thing with many, many humans.

The whole system of Natural Nutrition and Hair Hygiene is here for you to work with. No matter what your hair and scalp problem is, do not give up hope until you have given Mother Nature a chance to do her best to help you.

Those of you who have serious scalp and hair problems, just remember that it took you a long, long time to get that way . . . and it is going to take time for you to reverse the condition. Don't be impatient. Give Nature a chance to help you improve your hair and scalp.

YOU MUST MAKE YOUR BODY OBEY

You must understand that the mind must control the body. If you want good health and healthy hair and scalp, you have to be the master of your body. It must not tell you what it wants to eat. *You must tell your body what it's going to get!*

You must see that all the hygienic principles of Hair Culture are obeyed by the body. The body is lazy! It wants no part of routine. But YOU, as the Commander who gives the orders, must make it follow a regular routine for healthy hair and scalp.

REGULAR REST PERIODS ARE IMPORTANT

The body tends to be lazy even when it comes to rest and relaxation. It slumps. Don't let your body fool you into believing that mere inactivity is relaxing or restful. An incorrect sitting or lying position can cramp your muscles, squeeze your lungs and heart, interfere with the circulation of your blood stream . . . and actually do you more harm than good.

Strange as it may seem, the best and most natural way to rest is to stretch out on your back on a hard, unyielding surface. This makes it possible for your muscles to create their own natural traction and stretch in a relaxing manner, while the rib cage expands allowing full intake of oxygen and ample room for your heart to pump life-giving nourishment throughout your body and cleanse your blood stream of accumulated wastes.

A Slant Board is ideal for this purpose. Tilt it at a comfortable angle and lie on your back with your head at the lower end. This reverses the pull of gravity which your blood stream has to counteract in a sitting or standing position, and allows the waste-laden blood to drain from your feet and legs into the heart for purification. It helps your heart send nourishing food and oxygen to your brain and head.

This is particularly important for hair and scalp health. In the normally erect position of the body, your hair and scalp are the "high Alps" to which the life-giving blood stream must climb. By lying on the Slant Board with your head at the low end, you give your blood the chance to feed your "hair soil" and nourish your scalp.

BE A "CLOUD WALKER"

You may accomplish the same result by lying flat on your back on the floor, with your buttocks against the wall and your legs extended upward against the wall. In this position you may become a "cloud walker" like my rickshaw man in Hong Kong. A lean, muscular man in his sixties, he has trotted thousands of miles pulling rickshaws since he was sixteen—yet his legs show no sign of varicose veins but are as strong, smooth and cleanly muscled as a man of twenty.

He told me that twice daily for 15 to 30 minutes he becomes a "cloud walker"—lying in the position just described, and massaging his legs with downward strokes from the ankle, using oil to make the massage smooth and easy.

This type of rest period is equally or even more important for the sedentary or inactive person as it is for the athletic or active man or woman. A couple of 5-to-10 minute rest periods of this type—your back flat on a hard surface, your legs extended upward—will help to renew your overall vitality . . . and be especially beneficial to your Hair and Scalp Health.

SLEEP—NATURE'S GREATEST RESTORER OF HEALTH

Sleep is one of the most powerful and vital processes that a human being can possibly engage in. Every move we make, every thought we think during our waking hours causes us to spend a certain amount of vitality, breaking down tissue and creating toxic wastes. During sleep the "action" cells are at rest, and the natural restorative forces of the body are at work . . . eliminating poisonous wastes and rebuilding broken down tissue in body and brain. It is during sleep that the Life Principle flows back into us ... that our loss of vitality is made good.

So wonderfully adjusted is this principle of restoration that our balance in the "Bank of Life" might at any time be computed by merely striking a balance between what we spend of our vitality during our waking life ... and what we regain of this during the night ... multiplied by the length of time we have kept up this pace.

As with everything else that affects your general health ... so the amount and quality of restorative sleep that you get is reflected in the condition of your hair and scalp. Loss of sleep can result in loss of hair or loss of its lustre. If the scalp is not cleansed of toxic poisons and the hair soil not renourished during sleep, your "Crowning Glory" will fade away.

Your hair mirrors the quantity and quality of your sleep. Sleep is the greatest "hair restorer" on the market—and it's free!

FOR HEALTHY HAIR—GET 8 HOURS OF RESTFUL SLEEP EVERY NIGHT

Isn't it miraculous that Mother Nature can rebuild and restore our vitality in just one-half the time we spend in tearing it down? We can accomplish much more and do it better in 16 hours of effort, followed by 8 hours of restorative sleep, than we ever can by squandering our energy to the point of exhaustion because of impatience to "finish something and get rid of it." What we are really "finishing" and "getting rid of" is our health! And one of the first evidences of this depletion shows in lifeless, unhealthy hair.

If you want a head of beautiful, strong, healthy hair eight hours of restful sleep every night is a "must."

Not just sleep—but RESTFUL SLEEP. Again you must take command of your lazy body, which often wants to fall asleep just any old way. Sleeping in a cramped position, or on too soft a mattress, or in such a way that the circulation is blocked ... is *not* restful sleep.

One should sleep on a firm mattress, or place a board under a soft one. This allows the muscles to stretch in natural relaxation, and relieves pressure on vital organs. If you have pains in the neck, try sleeping without a pillow. If you must use a pillow—use a soft baby pillow.

Never sleep with your head pressing on your arms. This can cause neuritis in the arms. Make sure that you do not cross limbs or rest your head on other parts of the body . . . as this hinders the circulation of the blood. And it is during sleep that the blood stream must flow freely to do its restorative work.

Don't take your worries to bed with you! The sayings "He worried himself bald" . . . or, "She worried herself gray" . . . are not without basis in fact.

To repeat, the quantity and quality of your hair reflect the quantity and quality of your sleep. When you brush your hair at night, brush away tangled thoughts as well. Both you and your hair will be glowing with life in the morning.

HOW TO BRUSH YOUR HAIR

Give yourself a health and beauty treatment while brushing your hair. Stand with feet wide apart, knees slightly bent, head forward and down below the heart level. This brings the blood flowing easily to the scalp, cleansing and nourishing the "hair soil" . . . and at the same time it will be helping to revitalize the tissues of your face and neck.

Brush with a downward stroke from scalp to hair tips. The gentle tug of the brush helps to stimulate and loosen the scalp, while the brushing sweeps out dirt as well as dead hairs and the natural flakes of dead skin from the scalp.

Long hair—for almost two centuries the prerogative of women, but now popular with young men as well—should be brushed away from the scalp strand by strand, under and over, a few inches at a time. This method distributes the hair more evenly and makes it easier to arrange, as well as enhancing the coiffure by overall smoothness and glossiness.

45

CHOOSE YOUR OWN COMB AND BRUSH CAREFULLY

Each member of a family should have his own comb and brush. The best combs are those with smooth, blunt teeth. If the teeth of a comb are too pointed, the scalp may become scratched. Metal and fine combs should not be used, as these —may tear or break the hair. The use of a fine comb on the silky hair and tender scalp of babies is particularly to be condemned. From a sanitary standpoint also, the smooth blunt-toothed comb is most easily cleaned.

The rows of bristles of the brush should be stiff . . . but not so stiff that they will injure the scalp when used vigorously. Metal bristles are likely to tear the hair and irritate the scalp and their use should be avoided. The best results may be obtained from the use of two brushes, one with stiff bristles for working off the scales and stimulating the scalp, and another with softer bristles for smoothing and glossing the hair—an ideal health and beauty combination.

DAILY SCALP MASSAGE NECESSARY

For healthy hair, massage of the scalp morning and evening should become just as much of a ritual as brushing teeth. It stimulates hair growth by causing a freshening rush of blood to the scalp, nourishing all tissues that have to do with the growth of the hair. It loosens the scalp generally and thus assures good circulation. This promotes the growth of the pad of "hair soil" under the scalp, preventing degeneration of the scalp and hair follicles.

Remember, it is when you lose the hair soil on the skull that baldness sets in. Never forget that good nutrition and good circulation are absolutely necessary to cultivate this soil. Once the soil pad is gone and the scalp rests on the bony skull, hair cannot grow. Hair must have its own body soil to grow on. It must be well nourished and the blood must circulate through it.

Many men start out in life with a good head of healthy hair. But they are indifferent or ignorant about nutrition and the care of the hair . . . and then we have the start of baldness

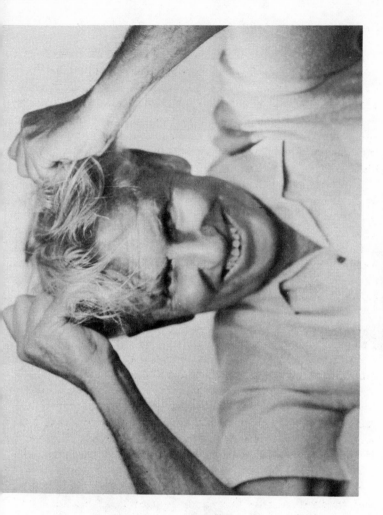

Pulling the hair improves circulation.

Now I see the secret of the making of the best persons, it is to grow in the open air, and eat and sleep with the earth.
—Walt Whitman

In health there is liberty. Health is the first of all liberties, happiness gives us the energy which is the basis of health.
—Miel

"Everything in excess is opposed by Nature."

—Hippocrates

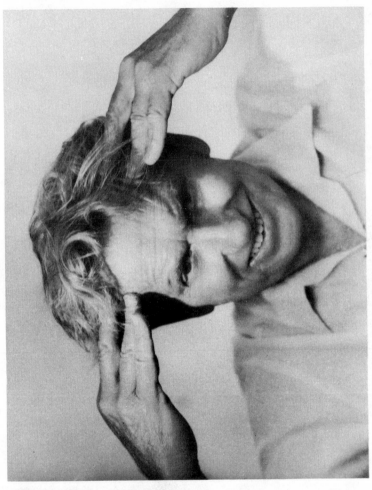

Simplicity...simplicity...simplicity, let your affairs be as two or three, and not as a hundred or a thousand.

The laws of health are inexorable; we see people going down and out in the prime of life simply because no attention is paid to them. —Bragg

Perfect health is above gold, and a sound body before riches. —Solomon

48

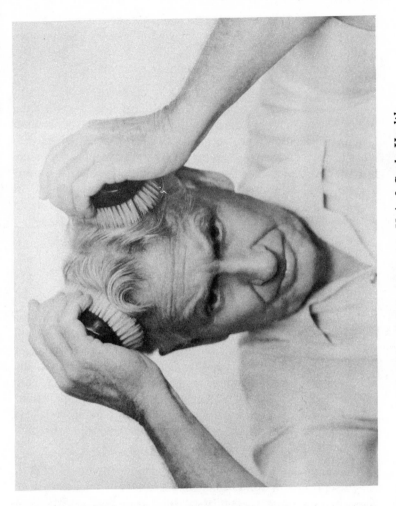

Brushing hair important to Hair & Scalp Health.

Whatsoever was the father of a disease; an ill diet was the mother.

—Herbert, 1859

Some students drink deeply at the fountain of knowledge—others only gargle.

and many other troubles of the hair and scalp. The hair must be cultivated exactly like a fine garden. It just will not take care of itself.

When good circulation in the scalp is assured by vigorous massage morning and evening, the glands of lubrication perform their functions more easily. This helps to loosen the scales and dirt, which are then easier to wash off.

Normal massage is not only a process of rubbing and kneading the scalp from front to back and from side to side, but also of pinching and pulling it from the underlying tissues, especially on the top and sides of the head where it is most firmly attached. Vibrating devices may be of some value, but they cannot be as effective as strong fingers deftly manipulated. The technique of scalp massage will be explained in detail later in this book, with illustrations showing how to give yourself a Self-Treatment for Hair and Scalp Health.

MASSAGE HELPS PREVENT BALDNESS

Along with proper nutrition the best preventive of baldness is daily massage of the hair. Unless falling hair is being caused by some internal disorder, massage is almost sure to help. As a matter of fact, there is hardly a single preparation on the market that does not enjoin its users to "rub into the scalp vigorously." Surely any persons who use such preparations must be aware of the fact that they are really being benefited by the rubbing rather than the sweet-smelling solutions they have poured on their heads.

Human nature being what it is, many people feel that if they spend money for a tonic they are helping the growth of their hair ... but that if they rub their heads with their fingers they are not getting anywhere. If the tonic does not contain harmful substances ... and does impel its user to massage his scalp when otherwise he would not bother ... it is serving a positive purpose in the care of the scalp.

DON'T BE AFRAID OF WATER ON YOUR HAIR!

It seems incredible that a legend should have developed discouraging the use of water in caring for the skin of the face, yet there are women who have definitely shunned water for years in favor of creams, lotions and astringents. The meaning of "aqua pura" is lost on these misinformed persons. The fact that water is the purest agent for ablutions seems absurd to their complicated reasoning. It is too easy to get!

There is no scientific proof that pure soap and water applied to the skin, hair and scalp is harmful. We have made wide research on this subject, and we cannot find a shred of evidence that the skin, hair and scalp can be harmed in any way by good soap and water. When we interviewed so-called "Skin, Hair and Scalp Specialists" who advocate the no-soap-and-water theory, we found that most of them have some preparation to sell for cleansing the skin, hair and scalp.

These manufacturers of skin and hair preparations have abetted this hygienic absurdity by claiming that their hair lotions occasionally will keep scalps clean and hair beautiful whether they are washed or not. Although the other parts of the body are washed thoroughly at least once a day, hair washing is often an infrequent rite attended with ceremony.

CLEANLINESS IS VITAL TO HAIR AND SCALP HEALTH

It is true that it is more difficult to keep the hair and scalp clean than perhaps any other part of the body. It requires time to wash the hair properly ... and time is the one commodity that moderns hate to expend. And yet hair holds dirt and impurities much more readily than do other parts of the body. In addition to external dirt, the hair retains the secretions of the oil and sweat glands and the scales of the scalp which are constantly being thrown off.

A normal scalp is extremely rare, and under modern conditions almost impossible to retain over any length of time. It is for this very reason that strict and regular care is imperative.

Unless one is willing to take the trouble necessary to keep the hair and scalp clean, one might just as well resign himself to irritations, infections and even ultimate loss of the hair. A clean scalp—or at least a scalp that is kept reasonably clean —is the basis of healthy, plentiful and beautiful hair. No artificial applications may help to bring about this condition unless there is a foundation of cleanliness and health.

In spite of the lure of bottled beauty, the simple but unromantic fact remains that THE ONLY WAY OF KEEPING THE HAIR CLEAN IS BY WASHING IT WITH GOOD SOAP AND WATER.

Washing never did and never will harm the hair. It does not dry the scalp. It does not destroy the hair growth. And it does not cause or increase dandruff. On the contrary, soap and water simply clean and do not lose their historic property when coming into contact with the scalp and hair.

Normally the scalp should be washed twice a week . . . but if infection is present, once a day is not too much. People with dry hair claim that washing is not good for it. The truth is that if they washed their hair more frequently, the scalp condition which causes dryness might have a chance to be cured. Cleanliness promotes health.

WHAT IS A SHAMPOO?

If the average person were asked what a shampoo is, the answer would probably be that it is a process of washing the hair and scalp. Most people who shampoo their own hair or have it shampooed have given little thought as to just what a shampoo really is, or what it can accomplish for the hair and scalp. They know that its effect is beneficial and pleasing, and that it should be done to keep their hair clean.

Every shampoo is really divided into two parts—washing the hair and washing the scalp. The old fashioned idea was that if the hair was clean, the scalp would take care of itself. This, however, is correct only as far as it goes . . . and because it is partly wrong, it is all wrong. Both the hair and the scalp must be thoroughly shampooed.

A SHAMPOO UNCLOGS YOUR SCALP

Underneath the skin of the scalp are the countless follicles of the hair. These take their nourishment from the blood. That is the reason we have gone into detail about building the proper blood to nourish the scalp. The hair and the scalp depend upon the kind of food you put into your body. We want you to remember that. Hair and scalp health begins with the food you eat. Live, vital foods build powerful heads of beautiful hair and healthy scalps.

As the flow of the blood in the scalp is normally sluggish, the underlying hair follicles do not always receive the vital nourishment they need from the blood. This is the reason for massage and manipulation which stimulates the flow of blood and exercises the skin. The increase in circulation provides an added supply of vital nourishment to the glands, and this results in helping you to have a healthy scalp and a fine growth of strong hair.

Each hair comes through one of the tiny pores in the skin. Obviously these pores must be kept clean, for if they are clogged with waste, dirt or dandruff the hair suffers . . . just as your complexion would suffer if you did not keep your face clean. A shampoo unclogs the pores.

A SHAMPOO MAKES YOUR HAIR SPARKLE

Now let us look at a hair. If you draw one of your own hairs through your fingers you will find that it is smooth when drawn one way and rough when drawn the other. Under a powerful microscope it can be seen that each hair is composed of tiny cells that overlap, like shingles on a roof. When the hair is perfectly clean, these little barbs project from the trunk of the hair, catching the light. This is the explanation of the sheen and lustre that clean, healthy, strong hair has.

Visualizing one hair with all these little projecting barbs, you will understand how dirt accumulates in the pockets at the base of the barbs where they join the trunk of the hair. When these minute pockets become filled with dust, dirt, grease, smog and other pollution from the air and foreign matter, the barbs can no longer reflect light and the hair loses its lustre and sheen. It becomes dull, dingy, lifeless, straw-like and unmanageable.

A proper shampoo cleans the hair itself, removing all the dirt, smog and grease from these pockets. Then the barbs stand out, catching the light and making the hair lustrous and bright—your "Crowning Glory."

MASSAGE AND BRUSH BEFORE SHAMPOOING

The hair and scalp should have their most vigorous workout before the shampoo. Start vigorous massage and manipulation with the hands pressed firmly upon the scalp. Move palm and fingers back and forth, up and down, with a circular motion . . . until every portion of the scalp is soft and flexible and moves freely.

Next you apply the stiff brushes to remove all of the dust, grease and dirt possible.

If your hair is quite oily, soak a piece of cotton in cider vinegar and with this saturate the entire scalp an hour before shampooing.

HOW TO SELECT YOUR SHAMPOO SOAP

The contents and the purity of the soaps to be used in washing the hair and scalp are of considerable importance. It would take an army of chemists to evaluate the various products on the market. There are a few general rules, however, which should be observed.

Soaps that are strong in alkali should never be used on the hair and scalp, because they not only remove the dirt and grease—but work on the tissue itself.

Besides alkali, the other principle content of soap is fat. If the fat is rancid it may cause irritation.

The cleansing properties of tincture of green soap are known to be especially good, but if used all the time it can be drying.

Generally speaking, most advertised shampoo creams and jellies act in the same way as ordinary soap.

For most scalps and hair, the ordinary neutral shampoo soaps of well known brands are as effective as expensive preparations, whether perfumed or medicated.

PURE CASTILE SOAP IS THE BEST. There is nothing better than a pure castile soap, shaved into water and dissolved over a slow fire. Never use a bar of soap rubbed directly onto the hair and scalp.

WASH HAIR AND SCALP IN SOFT WATER

The very best water in which to shampoo your hair is good natural rain water. It is worth the trouble to rig up a tank where you can catch plenty of rain water. A shampoo in rain water is the finest treatment your hair and scalp can receive. You should catch enough for shampooing, plus plenty more for drinking. Rain water is the finest of drinking water.

If you do not have rain water, the addition of sal-soda to the shampoo water will have a softening effect. Shampooing with hard water should be avoided unless a hard water soap is available.

HOW TO SHAMPOO THE HAIR CORRECTLY

Shampooing is in reality a combined chemical and mechanical action. The dirt, scales, grease and infectious matter are detached and washed away. The rules for proper shampooing are not complicated.

First, wet the hair with warm water. By wetting the hair before applying the shampoo soap, you protect it to some extent from any free alkali that may be in the soap.

Now apply the liquid soap. Start at the hairline in the front and work back, rubbing the soap in until it forms a thick sudsy lather, which should be kneaded into the scalp with the fingertips.

When you have been stricken by illness, your new car, your new home, your new big bank account—all these fade into unimportance until you have regained your vigor and zest for living again.—Peter J. Steincrohn, M.D.

Unless the hair is very dirty, greasy and oily, it is not necessary to use a brush in working in the lather, as a good shampoo can be given with the hands. Use your fingertips to scrub into the scalp and loosen the scales and the dirt. Remember we live in a polluted world. So much poison is floating around in the air, and it embeds itself into the hair and the pores of the scalp.

Continue the massaging of the scalp. Three soapings are usually necessary to thoroughly clean the scalp and hair.

RINSE HAIR THOROUGHLY

Rinsing should be thorough, because this is the process that actually carries the impurities from the hair. It should be continued until every trace of soap and dirt has been removed.

The notion that it is necessary to leave the soap in the hair for 10 or 15 minutes before rinsing, in order to "cut" out all the grease, is erroneous. Furthermore, if the lather remains in the hair too long it will probably dry out too much.

After the third soaping, give the hair and scalp two thorough rinses in warm water.

Follow this with a VINEGAR RINSE. Using 2 tablespoons of CIDER VINEGAR to a pint of warm water, pour the rinse over the hair and scalp. Thorough rinsing with the vinegar is essential, because particles of soap left in the hair will keep it from looking and feeling its best. It is the vinegar which "cuts" the soap and any remaining grease from the hair and scalp.

Finish off after the vinegar rinse with a cold water rinse. This stimulates circulation in the scalp, and at the same time closes the pores which have been opened and cleansed by the hot water.

When you can see little water crystals on the hair you will know that it has been thoroughly rinsed and is free from soap. Be sure that the hairline all around the head is given special attention as well as back of the ears.

It is time to dust off your dreams and shine up your ideas.

RINSE FOR BLONDES

If blondes use a vinegar rinse, only 1 tablespoon of vinegar should be used to a quart of warm water.

A LEMON RINSE is often preferred, as many blondes say that vinegar darkens their hair. The Lemon Rinse for blonde hair is made with the juice of 1 lemon strained into a pint of warm water.

This also should be followed with a cold water rinse.

DRY YOUR HAIR IN THE SUN

The best place to dry your hair (weather permitting) is out in the sunshine and fresh air. On cold days, if the sun shines into your home, stand or sit near a window and let the sun's rays dry your hair.

Mechanized heat is not recommended. It is usually too hot and after constant use makes the hair brittle. It is true that this is the quickest way to dry the hair, but it is not the best.

Your hair is a valuable asset to your personal appearance. Take time to wash and dry it correctly, so that your hair will be beautiful and feel good after shampooing.

A FEW EXTRA NOTES ON SHAMPOOING

We have found that shampooing under the shower is the simplest and the most effective method for cleansing both short and long hair. It is far more comfortable than bending over a basin, makes it easier to rinse the hair thoroughly and also to control the temperature of the water, and the force of the water from the shower stimulates circulation in the scalp.

Effective shampooing of the hair is as simple as we have described it. Refinements and the addition of homemade "secrets" usually add nothing, and may sometimes undo the good accomplished.

However, the time-honored custom of rubbing the white of an egg into the hair before shampooing, or adding it to the shampoo water, does sometimes increase the gloss of the hair and help to prevent dryness.

Unusual dryness of the scalp may also be helped by the

application of olive, almond, castor or coconut oil before the shampoo. It may even be applied the night before and the hair covered with a towel turban.

Some persons like to use a hair conditioner rinse after the vinegar or lemon rinse. There are many such preparations on the market. Since the hair conditioner penetrates only the outer layer of the hair it is usually harmless, and might rectify some of the damage caused by other commercial preparations (such as permanents, dyes, color rinses, etc.)

WASH YOUR COMB AND BRUSH, TOO

In a normal body the scalp and the hair will take adequate care of themselves if simply kept clean. As we have stated, castile soap and water are all that is required for cleansing purposes. Wash your hair whenever you think it needs it and that should be at least twice a week.

Before washing your hair, you should first wash both your comb and brush. Also keep hair curlers, clips, hair nets, etc., clean. There is little profit in cleansing your hair and scalp if you then work them over with a dirty comb and brush.

A stiff-bristled nail brush should be used for washing your comb to be sure that the dirt, scales and grease are removed between the teeth.

Brushes are more difficult to clean than combs. The maximum of cleanliness is obtained most easily with a brush whose bristle-holder may be removed and sterilized by boiling. However, if boiling softens the bristles, a thorough washing in hot soapy water with a few drops of ammonia added will do just as well. A stiff nail brush may also be used to scrub deposits of dirt, scales and grease from the base of the bristles.

THE VALUE OF SEA WATER ON THE HAIR AND SCALP

The beneficial effects of water on the hair and scalp extend even to sea water. In fact, because of the salts it contains, sea water has a definitely stimulating effect on the hair and scalp, just as it does on the rest of the skin.

The popular notion that salt water is harmful to the hair probably arose from the fact that salt water which dries on the hair leaves a dry, sticky feeling. This can be easily overcome if the hair and scalp are thoroughly rinsed with fresh water before the sea water dries.

Since bathing caps rarely give complete protection from water, women might just as well bathe without them if they do not mind the inconvenience and temporary untidiness of having wet hair in their faces. Certainly there is no scientific reason for using a cap when bathing in fresh water (except at public swimming pools where women are not permitted to swim without bathing caps). The tight constriction of the usual bathing cap impairs circulation.

The beautiful women of the South Seas have hair that many other women might envy, but it is difficult to imagine them pulling on bathing caps before they plunge into their favorite pools. The same goes for the men of the South Seas. Patricia and I have spent many months roaming the South Seas and we very rarely find a bald headed man.

MY SOUTH SEA ISLAND EXPERIENCE

South Sea Island people spend a great part of their lives in and on the sea, yet they retain a luxuriant growth of beautiful, healthy hair all their lives. Even the men and women in their eighties and nineties have thick, beautiful hair.

They spend so much time in both salt and fresh water that the scalp and hair is always clean. Also, they have a Hair Culture and Hair Care all their own, which includes rubbing in coconut oil and a great deal of scalp massage.

Remember, too, that these primitive people are not exposed to the foodless foods of civilization. They eat a natural diet which includes plenty of fresh vegetables, fruits, seaweeds and fish. As we have stated, Iodine is a valuable nutrient to the body chemistry. And seaweed and fish furnish an abundance of Iodine to the people of the South Seas.

I spent the entire year of 1933 in the South Sea Islands researching the health and nutrition of its people. Every day during my stay there I ate the seaweeds. At the end of the year I found that my hair was thicker, stronger and healthier than it had ever been in my entire life.

Since my South Sea Island Adventure I have consistently used seaweed in my daily diet. As noted earlier in this book, Health Food Stores carry seaweed in many forms—kelp powder which you can sprinkle over your raw and cooked foods to lend a tangy, delicious flavor; and seaweed tablets which may be taken daily. In whatever form you take it, you will be assured of getting your daily ration of the all important Iodine.

THE TRUTH ABOUT DANDRUFF

Because dandruff is the chief hobgoblin of both the patent medicine racketeer and the ethical scalp specialist, it is important that more than ordinary attention be given this much misunderstood and abused subject.

"Nine out of ten persons who seek treatment for baldness suffer from what they call dandruff." ... so writes one of our leading dermatologists in a chapter which he entitles: "Premature Baldness and Dandruff."

Now we do not deny that "it might be said" ... but we do say that it should not be said, for the simple reason that it is not true. Moreover, we assert that BALDNESS AND DANDRUFF ARE BY NO MEANS TWINS, nor even necessarily close associates.

It is truly unfortunate that for decades our scientific authors—not knowing the cause of "idiopathic" or common baldness—have taken refuge in such statements as the above. This same authority goes on to assert that dandruff is invariably the sign of an unhealthy scalp. Yet every general practitioner knows that at some time in every person's life excessive dandruff occurs. In most cases examination will reveal no disease whatever. The healthiest scalps will often be found shedding abnormal dandruff—and many diseased scalps are at times apparently free from it.

SEBORRHEA IS NOT DANDRUFF

Seborrhea is usually described in our textbooks as synonymous with dandruff. Just why they are considered to be identical or even necessarily related conditions, scientific investigation fails to demonstrate. We know that there is a constant peeling or renewing of the outer layer of the skin of the entire body which is thrown off in minute cells or scales. These dead and discarded cells, when they become detached from the scalp, are called dandruff.

Seborrhea, however, is a very different physiological process. It is a normal discharge of the oily material known as sebum, which is secreted and exuded by the sebaceous glands. These glands are very numerous on the scalp and nose, and it is the discharge from them that causes the nose to appear oily or "shiny." To the scalp and hair the sebaceous glands supply the oil that produces the natural lustre and pleasant, silky softness to the hair.

Special attention is now directed to one of the smallest and most interesting of the body's muscles. It is called the arrector-pili muscle, which is the only muscle on the crown of the head. It is connected to each hair and the adjacent tissue and its action is involuntary and uncontrollable. This little muscle not only causes the hair to rise or "stand on end" or forms "goose flesh" ... but its contraction also expels the contents of the sebaceous glands.

Through some nerve impulse the arrector-pili muscle contracts and causes the oily white and yellowish contents of these little sacs, the sebaceous glands, to be constantly discharged. For some undetermined reason this discharge is more copious in some persons than in others. There is no known means of increasing or diminishing the flow.

To my mind the greatest mistake a person can make is to remain ignorant when he is surrounded, every day of his life, by the knowledge he needs to grow and be healthy and successful. It's all there. We need only to observe, read, learn ... and apply.

61

FREQUENT SHAMPOOING IS GOOD
FOR THE HAIR AND SCALP

Some men and women must shampoo the hair every day or every few days because of the oily build-up.

We knew a woman who had to shampoo her hair every day of her life on account of the heavy oily build-up. As we have stated, washing the hair and scalp with good castile soap never did any harm, regardless of how often it is done. Good soap and water are good for the hair and scalp.

"DRY" AND "OILY" DANDRUFF—BOTH NATURAL

Remember that dandruff and seborrhea result from two distinctly different processes, both of which are normal and natural. *Dandruff* is the exfoliation or shedding of the outer dead cells of the skin, which are normally moist. *Seborrhea* is the discharge of sebum from the sebaceous glands. The terms have been confused for centuries, for lack of intelligent observation.

The process resulting in what is called dandruff on the scalp is one which occurs all over the body—first, for purposes of renewal; secondly, to assist in the process of healing. Without this ability to slough off the outer dead layers of skin there would be no healing of the skin following such injuries as cuts, burns and scalds. So we see that the process which produces dandruff is an essential one.

In the case of persons whose scalps secrete a profuse amount of sebum or oil, the excess oil combines with the minute skin flakes to produce what is commonly known as "oily dandruff." In other cases, in which the skin exfoliation is heavy and the exudation of oil scanty, the product is the so-called "dry dandruff."

In either case, there is nothing pathological about the matter. Aside from the social annoyance there is nothing to be feared from either "oily" or "dry" dandruff. And one thing you may depend upon, notwithstanding all the pseudo-scientific nonsense to the contrary: DANDRUFF HAS NOTHING TO DO WITH BALDNESS.

Certain scalp "experts" exploit the fact that oils, soaps, special shampoos and antiseptics, combined with salves and water, and frequently applied, will cause a temporary removal of the surface scales called dandruff. But as the effects of these concoctions also depend upon Nature and her solicitude for her creations, the effects are fleeting or even absent. For the dead cells are constantly forming and falling in accordance with the requirements of Nature. Hence some "hair specialists" urge frequent use of their nostrums in order to conceal the natural process.

We find dandruff on persons of all ages and both sexes. Since women have it as well as men and children as well as adults, it is strange that it does not cause baldness in the case of young and healthy men.

Pitiful are the methods to which some "hair specialists" resort in order to make a case against dandruff!

DANDRUFF IS NON-INFECTIOUS

Some authors have gone so far as to assert that dandruff is infectious or contagious. The truth is that dandruff not only is non-infectious, but it actually has some slight antiseptic qualities. When the scalp is infected or injured by foreign bacilli, Nature's first defense move is usually to exude an abnormal amount of sebum . . . and scalp infections or injuries are thus often overcome without medical aid. The invading destructive germs are simply surrounded by the abnormal exudation of sebum . . . then the outer layer of skin is sloughed off as usual and the infectious organisms are carried away with it.

You need have no fear of "contracting" dandruff from the scalp of any person. It simply cannot be done . . . no more than you can contract disease from the fingernail or toenail parings of another person.

HAIR AND SCALP CARE WILL KEEP DANDRUFF MOVING OUT

The Program of Hair and Scalp Care as outlined in this book will show you how to keep dandruff from accumulating.

The first thing to remember is that the hair and scalp need a daily workout. The scalp must be vigorously massaged twice daily ... if not, the dandruff is going to cling to the scalp and to the hair itself.

Not only do you massage the scalp ... you grip the hair in your hands and vigorously move the scalp from side to side and then forward and backward ... then use a circular motion until every portion of the scalp is soft and flexible and moves freely.

For those people who have thin hair, the gripping and pulling of the hair should be postponed until the scalp has been loosened up by finger massage or a hand vibrator.

We have found in our long experience in Hair and Scalp Care that people who have tight scalps have hair and scalp problems. All forms of scalp and hair manipulation are decidedly useful, especially where the scalp does not move freely on the skull. Once the scalp is loosened, vigorous massage, pinching, kneading and gentle but firm pulling of the hair improves its strength and stimulates its growth.

Unfortunately, most people have grossly neglected the care of the scalp and hair, because most of them have not been told how very important it is to give attention to the hair and scalp. Then the hair starts to go and scalp problems begin to come.

From today on YOU can start to create a strong, healthy head of hair and a healthy scalp!

A FRANK AND HONEST DISCUSSION OF BALDNESS

Among the more important sacrifices of the human race in its evolution from the primitive to the civilized man, is the loss of hair as it grows on the head for adornment. Hottentots and Australian Bushmen do not suffer from baldness. When the African headhunters go out on a foraging expedition they bring back truly healthy heads of hair.

From time to time, however, some primitive people shave their heads to subscribe to the prevailing fashion note of the jungle. This in itself indicates that an abundance of hair is common and the lack of it unusual. So by artificially removing their hair the primitive man becomes "different" and exceptionally stylish.

Baldness, or alopecia, means simply the loss of hair. Whether it is only a slight thinning out or a complete absence of hair, whether it occurs only on the scalp, in other places, or over the whole body, it is still baldness.

BALDNESS NOT A SIGN OF BRAINS

To repeat, baldness is a condition almost entirely confined to civilized races. It is rarely found among primitive people who eat a natural diet and live an open-air life. This fact is probably responsible for the idea that baldness is a sign of unusual mental powers.

The lack of hair has nothing to do with the presence of brains, of course. The grain of truth in this notion is that intellectual people are more apt to lead sedentary lives and are otherwise not of good general physique. As a type they are highstrung and nervous, with a tendency to derangements of the glands of internal secretion. The tension, stress and strain of modern life produce constitutions so weak in powers of resistance that diseases of the scalp such as baldness are more easily contracted and more difficult to throw off. Thus, while not all bald heads are intellectual ... there are, as one writer has remarked, more bald heads to be seen at big business meetings than at a burlesque show.

HOW ARTIFICIAL HEAT AND LIGHT AFFECT THE HAIR

We have found in our investigations on baldness that living in artificially heated and cooled rooms may have something to do with baldness.

In New York City we visited a big Insurance Company where several hundred men were working at their desks in an enormous room, entirely under artificial lights. There was absolutely no daylight in the room. There were no windows. In the winter the room was heated artificially, and in the summer artificially cooled. At no time during their 8-hour day in this large room did these men get natural daylight or natural air.

Their ages ranged from 22 to 64. On actual count, more than half of them were completely or partially bald. Out of the 200 men we counted, only about 14 had good heads of healthy hair.

This was not an isolated case. We visited other large offices where the same conditions prevailed and found about the same condition of the men's hair. We also visited large offices where as many as several hundred women were working under the same artificial conditions, and found some poor hair and scalp conditions among them.

The hair and scalp need sunlight and fresh air. People who are forced to work under artificial lights and breathe artificial air should make it a point every day to give their hair and scalp a sun and air bath. Spend your lunch hour in a park, letting your hair and scalp have the refreshment of sunshine and fresh air while you enjoy your picnic health lunch. Your entire body will benefit. The men and women whom we saw working under artificial conditions had pale faces. Their ears were pale and their lips lacked that redness that comes from fresh air and sunlight.

DOES CLIMATE AFFECT BALDNESS?

In our research on baldness we have heard it said that extremes of temperature are detrimental to the propagation and perpetuation of the hair. Some people say that hair thrives best in a temperate climate, neither too warm nor too cold. Others add that climate must not be too dry or too humid.

Well, we thoroughly investigated this hypothesis also. We found that among the Laplanders, who live in the cold ... and the tropical peoples, who live in the heat ... baldness is very uncommon. Among the civilized peoples of the temperate zones, it flourishes.

SHALL WE BLAME HEREDITY FOR BALDNESS?

Most bald people blame their baldness on heredity. In order to give this heredity thesis any status, we must first answer the question why women very seldom inherit baldness, although they have the same kind of scalps, cranial structure and hair growing properties as men. There is a tendency to escape this dilemma by saying that baldness is a secondary sexual characteristic of the male. But secondary sexual characteristics, when they truly exist, are common to all men and not limited to a minority as is simple baldness. And why do not brothers always share equally in this inheritance? That they do not is commonly known.

WHAT OUR WORLDWIDE RESEARCH REVEALS

Traveling as we do all over the world we have the opportunity to study whether heredity is the real cause of baldness. We know a family in Australia on a large sheep station (we would call it a ranch in the United States). There are nine brothers living and working together on the station. Six of them have perfect heads of hair. Three are almost bald. Their ages range from 30 to 50. The father, who is in his seventies, has been bald since his early twenties. Their mother has a normal head of hair.

It has been stated by some hair and scalp authorities that highly nervous men are prone to baldness. But on investigation we found this not to be true. In mental hospitals and insane asylums, both here and abroad, it has been shown that there is no greater percentage of baldness among patients of these institutions than among other segments of society.

WHAT CAUSES BALDNESS?

Now we are going to give our opinion on baldness. We will begin by saying that all the cells, organs, bones and tissues of the body are fed by the blood stream ... and that all these cells depend for their health upon the quality of the nourishment that the blood carries to them. If the blood is deficient in some important nutrient that is needed to build a certain kind of cell, that cell is going to suffer from malnutrition.

First, we believe that a good head of hair begins at conception. When a new life is started in the womb of the mother, that new baby gets its nourishment from the mother. If the mother does not get the essential nutrients to build a healthy body soil for the unborn baby's hair . . . then sooner or later in that new human's life the deficiency is going to show.

Let's say that a child is born with a tendency to weak, thin hair . . . and that after it is born, it is still not getting the full daily rations of important nutrients to build a strong head of hair. Incorrect prenatal feeding on the part of the mother while carrying the child and inadequate nutrition during the child's early life gives the individual a difficult start on an unbalanced health foundation. We can state it this way—baldness is most often the tragedy of poor nutrition, along with faulty hair and scalp habits.

You may ask, "If in your opinion you feel that baldness is due to a nutritional problem, why is it that in the same family there will be baldness in some males and not in others?" . . . as in the Australian family mentioned previously.

We must answer the question this way. Every human is a chemical laboratory and each works differently. Some humans have or are born with a better chemical laboratory than others, and have the power to convert certain foods to certain chemicals. Each one of us is different, just as each snowflake and oak leaf has a different pattern. You must remember you are YOU! There has never been anyone made exactly like you and there never will be.

HOW CAN SCIENTIFIC NUTRITION HELP BALDNESS?

We are not saying that proper nutrition is the cure for baldness. We have no cures for baldness. But we have seen some interesting things happen through scientific nutrition to people who were bald. These people had read our books or attended our Health Lectures.

THE CASE OF MR. S. OF NEW YORK CITY

In 1956 we gave a series of Health Lectures in New York City. Remember these were lectures on the effect of scientific nutrition on the human body. We made no claims for cures of any kind. Our message was and is that better nutrition is bound to make better humans. This important fact is certainly not disputed by animal breeders, who are trained specialists in the proper feeding of animals to make them healthier and more saleable. We feel that human beings are more valuable, and see no reason why they should not enjoy the benefits of scientific nutrition.

As elsewhere, our students in New York got a thorough education in scientific nutrition and applied this knowledge to their own bodies. We asked for no personal testimonials. We never do—but over the years we have received thousands from people who attend our lectures and read our books.

In 1960—four years after we gave our class in scientific nutrition in New York—Mr. S. sent an unsolicited testimonial telling us how he had gained healthy weight and no longer had a thin, weak body. By following our teachings he was now enjoying superior health.

"When I took your class I was 43 years of age and had lost most of the hair on top of my head," he wrote. "But within the last year I see hair again growing on my head, which I credit to my improved good health through scientific nutrition."

Again in 1965 Mr. S. wrote, telling us that he had resumed his game of handball which he had not played for many, many years due to LACK OF ENERGY. He told us how happy he was because he could now part his healthy hair.

Mr. S.'s correspondence is similar to the numbers of other unsocilited letters which we receive from our students all over the English speaking world.

Now learn what and how great benefits a temperate diet will bring with it. In the first place, you enjoy good health—Horace, 65-8 B.C.

YOU ARE WHAT YOU EAT

In our lecture and class work we teach the care and hygiene of the hair as given in this book. We promise no miracles. We promise no cures. We simply say, "You are what you eat." To build a strong, healthy body you must feed your body the important nutrients that it requires for perfect functioning. To have a good, healthy scalp and hair, you must feed them properly.

We sincerely wish that we could promise every person with a hair or scalp problem the benefits that Mr. S. received from proper nutrition. But that we cannot do. *We can only help you to help yourself!* And that is as far as we can go.

We feel that PREVENTION is the one great service we can render to our students. The time to feed your body correctly for a full head of hair is while you have hair on your head. It is then that it should be guarded and massaged and carefully groomed. Do not wait until it is gone and then ask for miracles to happen.

KEEP HEALTHY FOR LUXURIANT HAIR

We sincerely believe that good health and proper nutrition are vitally important in having a good head of strong, healthy hair. Now while you have it is the time to take care of it.

Our search for the causes of baldness and other scalp and hair problems goes on day after day. We would like to know exactly what is the cause of baldness and how it can be remedied. Not just a few isolated causes—but something from which every bald person could get results. As it stands this minute, we feel that nutrition plays an important role.

Again we say to the person who has his or her hair ... treasure it and take extra special care of it.

MEN'S HATS MAY BE A CAUSE OF BALDNESS

We, the authors of this book, have traveled all over the world and have had a chance to observe thousands of bald headed men. Among men who get a balanced diet and do not wear hats we see the least amount of baldness. Good nutrition and free circulation of the blood to the scalp certainly have a great deal to do with men keeping their hair.

The hair depends upon a good supply of rich, red blood carrying plenty of oxygen. The great pipes that carry the blood to the hair are called the temporal blood vessels. 98% of all men's hats press on the temporal arteries and veins and restrict the flow of blood to the hair and scalp.

If the hair suffers from interference with the temporal blood supply, the scalp itself—which also depends upon these blood vessels—suffers equally. It will invariably be found that the scalp of the bald man is abnormal in the area covered by the hat. Below the hat band, however, the scalps of both the bald and the non-bald will be found not to differ appreciably. Look at the men around you, and you will find many of them bald on the top or crown of the head but with a good growth of hair below the hat band.

During the last ten years we have been studying the construction of men's hats all over the world. Practically all of them compress the frontal temporal artery and vein. The frontal temporal vein and artery are located on the right side of the head, on a line with the tip of the lobe of the right ear. (NOTE: In a following section of this book you will learn how to stimulate this area with scalp massage to increase the blood circulation into the scalp and hair.)

Since the hat is often the worst offender, it might seem that the simplest preventive measure would be for men to stop wearing hats. But the problem is not so simple as that. There are thousands of men in military service, as well as railroad workers, bus and taxi drivers, airplane pilots—and in hundreds of other employments—who are required to wear uniforms and hats while on duty. Practically all these hats compress the frontal temporal vein and artery. Above all others, these men who are forced through necessity to wear hats, should follow the daily program of scalp and hair massage (described and illustrated on following pages) which will open up these important blood vessels.

THE HAIR AND SCALP NEED GOOD CIRCULATION

The hair and scalp need oxygen. Going without a hat gives the ventilation needed by the hair and scalp. We find that most people who are habitually hatless have excellent hair.

However, it does not necessarily follow that wearing a hat destroys the hair—except those hats which fit too tightly about the temples, compressing the blood vessels and cutting off the blood supply. As noted above, this pressure also tends to starve the layer of "soil" that provides the scalp and hair with nourishment.

Tightly fitting, unventilated felt hats for men and women are also harmful, because they increase perspiration which irritates the scalp and lays it open to infection. The same applies to tight bathing caps—buy them extra large.

Parents of children whose heads are broadest at the temples would do well to dispense with the present form of hats, and insist upon securing hats made to bridge over and protect the temporal vein and artery.

All humans would be better off if they discarded hats. We realize, however, that this is not possible. In colder climates and among people of poor health and weak constitutions it is impractical to dispense with hats ... and, as stated above, some people are forced by their employment to wear hats. And some prefer to wear them. But everyone who wears a hat should make sure that it does not restrict the flow of blood to the hair and scalp.

TEACH THE RULES OF HAIR HEALTH TO CHILDREN

The time to prevent baldness is before it starts. Most men wait until they start getting bald before they do anything about it.

Children should be taught early in life about the danger of permanent baldness, and trained to follow a good Program of Health and Hair Hygiene which they can continue throughout life. If the Program as outlined in this book were practiced among parents and their children, it is our opinion that within twenty years there would surely be fewer bald heads.

USE THIS SELF-TREATMENT TO KEEP
YOUR HAIR AND SCALP HEALTHY
AND HELP PREVENT BALDNESS

In closing this discussion, we should mention that although baldness usually begins at the front of the upper cranium and progresses slowly backward, this is not always the case. When the hair begins to fall first—not at the front—but at the back, we know that the posterior temporal blood vessels have been affected first. The following illustrated section shows you how to massage these posterior temporal blood vessels as well as the frontal temporal vein and artery.

Before beginning your self-treatment, simple though it is, study carefully the course of your temporal blood vessels. They run up to your head immediately in front of your ears, and very close to the surface of the skin. You can trace them very easily with the fingertips.

Use your fingers and apply pressure firmly and evenly, but gently. Always follow the course of the blood vessels, and never use a circular movement. Avoid rubbing the blood vessels crosswise.

CAUTION: To wear a hat that exerts pressure on the temporal veins and arteries defeats the object of this treatment.

For the first three months it would be well to employ this treatment twice daily, upon rising and before retiring. For complete illustrated details of the Self-Treatment study the following pages.

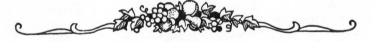

. . . *Of the complete protein foods, the egg has the highest biological value. Gram for gram it has the most ability to support life. The egg (fertile is best − Ed.) also has a larger proportion of the amino acid methionine than any other complete protein. Methionine is one of the amino acids which has been found useful in stimulating hair growth.*
− John J. Carella

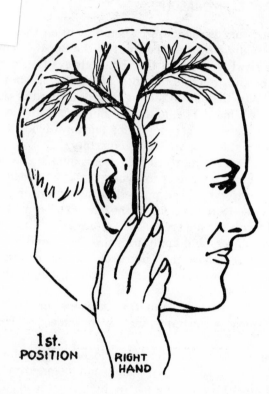

1st.
POSITION   **RIGHT**
HAND

Place the palm-side of the tips of the first three fingers of your right hand gently but firmly over the temporal artery and vein on the right side of your head, on a line level with the tip of the lobe of your right ear. (The illustration above shows the correct position.)

Now glide the fingers, exerting slight pressure, upwards to a point an inch or so above the top of your ear (or just below the point at which your hat-band normally contacts your head.)

This motion "squeezes" the blood upward through the temporal artery toward the scalp.

74

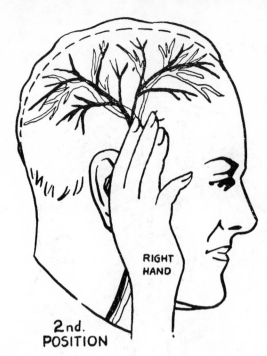

RIGHT
HAND

2nd.
POSITION

THEN . . .

Maintain the position of your right hand, so holding the fingers as to prevent the blood from returning. (See the illustration above.)

There are a number of reasons why one may suffer from poor blood circulation. Many are related to diet and nutrition. A deficiency in any one of the vitamins or minerals necessary for the maintenance of our health may lead to restricted circulation. Cholesterol deposits which affect the major arteries and veins of the body may also affect the smaller blood vessels of the scalp. Nervous tension, which very well may be the result of a nutritional deficiency, may cause a reduction in the amount of blood reaching the area of the scalp . . .

There are also physical reasons why one may have restricted circulation. Most women have wider blood vessels than men. This may be a partial explanation for the fact that more men lose their hair than women . . . Improper diet for an extended period can aggravate this situation (a tight scalp). A tight scalp does not necessitate the loss of hair. One with such a condition will have to place more emphasis on scalp massage than others, in addition to the recommended dietary actions.

– John J. Carella

75

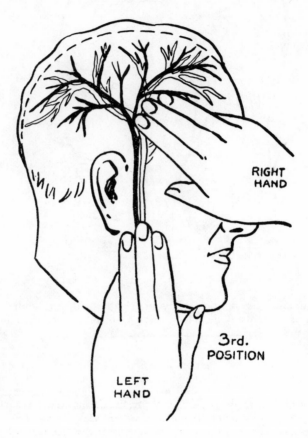

RIGHT
HAND

3rd.
POSITION

LEFT
HAND

NOW . . .

Still maintaining the position of your *right* hand, start the palm
side of the first three fingers of the *left* hand upward until they
touch the fingertips of your *right* hand, "squeezing" gently upward
just as you did with your right hand. (The illustration above
shows how.)

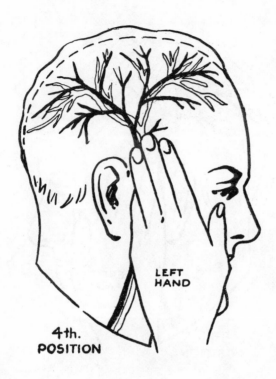

LEFT HAND

4th. POSITION

NOW . . .

Release your right hand, but maintain the position of your left hand (see illustration) and repeat the "squeezing" motion of your right hand. Then left again, maintaining the position of your right hand at the top of the "pressure area." Repeat these motions, always commencing pressure below before releasing pressure above.

NOW . . .

Repeat the motions described above several times. Then finish the last upward stroke with your *left* hand, and *hold* it as the top position. Your left hand will then be holding the blood in the scalp as pictured in illusration No. 4, compressing the temporal artery and vein just below the hat-band location.

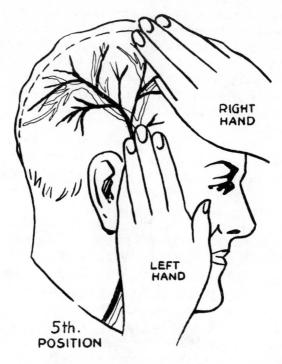

RIGHT
HAND

LEFT
HAND

5th.
POSITION

NOW *(and most importantly)*

Still maintaining the position of your left hand as stated above, place the palm-side of the same three fingertips of your right hand at a point midway between the center of the top of your head and the position of your left fingers. The illustration above shows the correct position.

Then, commence pressure from above, moving the fingers of your right hand downward over the skull until the fingers of both hands meet.

THEN . . .

Repeat these operations exactly, starting, however, with the left hand, on the temporal region of the left side of your head.

THE NEW HAIR TRANSPLANT OPERATION FOR BALDNESS

Today great advances have been made in surgery. The one of particular interest here was developed by Dr. Norman Orentreich, clinical research dermatologist, who worked out a technique for dissecting growing hair from the back of the scalp and transplanting it to bare bald spots of the head.

Recently I heard a well known T. V. commentator express great satisfaction as to the results of such transplant surgery in his case. It was absolutely amazing what this operation had done for this man. Hair is now growing where there was once only a bald spot.

It has been reported that thousands of men have benefited from this new transplant surgery, and that the technique has been developed into a simple office procedure. Bald people should investigate this new operation. It may be your answer to baldness.

SHOULD MEN AND WOMEN WEAR WIGS TO CONCEAL BALDNESS?

In today's world we are judged by others to a large extent by our personal appearance. Most people look at us and evaluate us solely on what they see.

The people in the entertainment field know this—and many, many stars of stage, screen, T.V. and night clubs wear wigs or specially made hairpieces to cover bald spots.

We say definitely that if wearing these added hairpieces or wigs is going to improve your appearance and make you feel more youthful and self-confident, then by all means go to a good hair specialist and have him create exactly what you want in the way of hair. If it will raise your morale, then by all means do it at once.

THE PROBLEM OF GRAY HAIR

When gray hair starts to show, no one wants it. A woman, peering into the mirror above her dresing table, discerns a gray hair among her brown. She sighs profoundly. Her first gray hair! Immediately she experiences, kaleidoscopically, the whole seeming tragedy of age—one by one the disappearance of her charms and the eventuality of the beckoning grave. A man, while shaving, notices a few white hairs at his temple. His razor stops short in the air. Dismayed, he examines his hair. This is the climax—this is dignity and the end of fun. No matter how philosophical these two persons may become in time, their first thoughts are filled with sorrow and pity for themselves.

THE BIG QUESTION

Should the lady or gentleman, brooding on their misfortune, happen to see the promises of a "color restorer" in an advertisement, they become easy prey to the advertised suggestion: "Why have unsightly gray hair?"

Why, indeed—unless gray hair is really not unsightly ... unless, as a matter of fact, it may be truly beautiful when not subjected to experimental treatment? Perhaps "unsightly" as an adjective applied to gray hair was the figment of a dye manufacturer's imagination. Playing on the human fear of age, the nostalgia of growing older, he added the fear of looking ugly.

Unless men and women are professional persons, the color of whose hair must remain static in the interest of their careers ... or unless their daily breadwinning positions depend upon deceiving employers as to their true age ... there is no reason why the charlatanism of hair dyeing should receive the support of an anxious public. It is questionable which is more unsightly—a person whose hair is gray, or that same person with ill-concealed dyed hair and the risk of developing skin diseases or internal disorders from the metallic or aniline contents of the preparations used. No better application could be made of La Rochefoucauld's penetrating observation:

> *The ordinary employment of artifice is the mark of a petty mind; and it almost always happens that he who uses it to cover himself in one place, uncovers himself in another.*

80

DON'T BE BRAINWASHED INTO DYEING

The hair dye manufacturers have done a tremendously good job of brainwashing people who are beginning to turn gray or have already become so. On the T.V. screen you see this brainwashing in action, especially for women.

This particular T.V. commercial appeared recently: Sitting dejected in the corner of her living-room was a wife who was starting to turn gray. In the same room her husband (with gray hair) was reading his paper, paying absolutely no attention to his wife. Then you heard her speak her thoughts aloud, saying, "He no longer loves me. I no longer attract my husband because I am too old looking with this ugly gray hair."

Then she picks up a magazine and eagerly reads a hair dye advertisement that tells her a woman's life can instantly be changed by dyeing her hair . . . years are rolled back and lover boy husband will see her as he saw her before marriage. So the "little woman" dashes out and purchases a glamorous hair dye.

Now the magic wand has been waved. Her husband no longer reads his newspaper, but concentrates all his attention on his wife. He is shown bringing her flowers and presents and taking her out dancing.

What utter nonsense! As if the color of the hair would change a man and wife's emotional life. True love is not turned off and on with hair dye.

NO KNOWN MEANS OF "RESTORING" NATURAL COLOR

We wish we had the answer to gray hair. Several years ago Dr. Alice Morgan, of the University of California at Berkeley, announced to the world that by feeding massive doses of B Complex Vitamins to aging minks she was able to change their gray hair back to its original dark color. She did not state that it would do the same for humans. Nevertheless, thousands of gray haired people started to take B Complex Vitamins. Here and there we would find a person who told us that this treatment had turned their gray hair back to its natural color.

To date, no physiological or internal process is known which makes it possible to alter the color of white or gray hair. In other words, there is no such thing as "restoring" the natural color of hair.

WHAT CAUSES GRAY HAIR?

In our opinion it is not a matter of "growing old." Because you do not grow old. There is no cell in your body that is over eleven months old. So what is there to grow old? There is degeneration of the human body, but years do not make you older in this way. There are many people in their seventies and eighties who show on physical examination that biologically they have the organs of a person half their calendar years ... and a person of thirty may well prove on physical examination to have a biologically aging body. Every day you see prematurely old people ... and old people who remain young.

Let's take for example the great actress Gloria Swanson. This elegant, glamorous, beautiful lady admits to being in her late seventies. Yet she is a beautiful person. She is biologically young. We have seen women half her calendar years who show more signs of premature aging.

AGE IS NOT TOXIC

So get it out of your mind that birthdays make you old and gray. Age is not toxic. You bring on premature aging by the way you feed yourself and the care you give your body.

You must remember that *the most permanent thing in life is change*. Your body is in a state of constant change every second of your life by a ceaseless motion of chemical activity. From the minute you arrive on this earth changes begin to take place in your body.

Grayness, however, is gradual. It is a sign of maturity. It generally shows first on the temples, then spreads to the crown and the rest of the head.

NATURE'S COLORING PROCESS

The color of the hair depends upon the middle or cortical layer of the hair, which consists of cells containing an oily fluid with minute grains of pigment and sometimes bubbles of air. The color of the hair is determined by the color of the grains of pigment, and the exact shade by the quantity of these grains in the fluid. A density of grains will produce a dark shade. If the grains are scarce, the hair will be lighter in tone. Air bubbles also serve to lighten the shade.

According to researchers who have devoted a great deal of time to studying the pigmentation of the hair, there are only two main colors of pigment granules—reddish yellow and sepia brown—whose combinations or diffusions produce all the shades which we commonly see. When the reddish yellow granules are thick in the cortical fluid and the air cells are scarce, the color of the hair is a bright red. If the sepia brown pigments are present but diffused by the air cells, the hair color is light yellow. Thence it deepens to dark brown and black, depending upon pigment density. The two types of pigment may be combined to produce a variety of intermediate shades.

One interesting result of this research was the conclusion that there is no such thing as coal-black hair. No black pigment was found in the hairs of Chinese, Japanese, Indians or Negroes. In every case it was the dense formation of the sepia brown pigment that produced apparent blackness.

Scattered throughout the loose structure of the cortical layer are cells which hold air and oil from the sebaceous glands. This oil helps to hold the pigment in suspension and prevents the coloring fluid from drying up or evaporating.

WHAT HAPPENS TO MAKE HAIR TURN GRAY?

For some unknown reason the bodily functions which produce the oil fluids containing the hair's coloring matter will in time slow up or cease. The oils begin to dry up and the grains of pigment gradually disappear, air bubbles taking their place and appearing as tiny spots of white or whitish yellow along the hair shafts. Under the microscope this appears as a mottled hair, but to the naked eye as a gray hair. When all the pigment is gone and the air bubbles are still more numerous, the hair becomes white.

GRAY HAIR CAN BEGIN AT ANY AGE

We have met thousands of young men and women in our travels over the world and have found boys and girls as young as fourteen years turning gray. On the other hand we have met people who have reached the age of ninety without a gray hair in their heads. While we were lecturing in New Zealand last year, for example, we met a gentleman in his early nineties who had a full head of strong, beautiful, naturally colored brown hair. While we were in London, we met a lady of ninety-two whose lovely head of hair showed no trace of gray.

Yet some of the finest specimens of young manhood and womanhood that we have met were turning gray or completely so. As far as we know today, there is no answer as to why some people lose the pigmentation in their hair so much earlier than others.

DON'T BE AFRAID OF GRAY HAIR

I noticed the first gray hair creeping in around my temples in my late fifties. Knowing that the most permanent thing in life is change, I welcomed my new coloring. In fact, to my way of thinking, gray hair softens the features of the maturing person.

These gray hairs did not slow down my physical or my mental activities in any shape, manner or form. I do not consider gray hair a sign of old age, nor do I think it is ugly or unsightly.

I see many of my male friends who are frightened about their gray hair, so they use all kinds of dyes to disguise it. I have no argument with those who want to dye their hair. This is a personal decision and up to each individual. My home is in Hollywood, California, and I have been Diet and Physical

Culture Consultant to some of the most highly paid and successful film and T.V. stars for the past fifty years. Many of these people meet the graying of their hair in panic. So they dash off and get their hair dyed. Not only members of the theatrical profession, but men and women in other walks of life cannot reconcile themselves to having gray hair, so they get it dyed. Fine, I say. If that makes them feel younger and look younger, I'm all for hair dyeing.

INVESTIGATE BEFORE YOU DYE YOUR HAIR

Just remember that when you have dye on your hair you are taking a calculated risk. To me personally the inadvisability of using hair dyes is apparent even before they are applied. A successful dye must penetrate between the scales of the hair cuticle to deposit color on the cortex of the hair shaft. The use of hair dyes must be carefully supervised since a slightly overbalanced proportion may result in destroying not just the oil, but the entire hair.

Most dangerous because they are less obvious are the injuries to general health which may be caused by the presence of poisonous substances in the dye which are absorbed through the skin.

Dermatologists are constantly confronted with cases of poisoning from dyes with a metallic base. Such dyes usually contain chemical solutions of such metals as silver, mercury, tin, lead, bismuth, etc. Our opinion is that these are dangerous. The harmful effects may be noticed soon after application, or the poisons may be absorbed more slowly and the toxic symptoms may not appear for some time, depending upon individual susceptibility. Sometimes there will be no apparent ill effect for many years except an excessive dryness of the hair.

TO DYE OR NOT TO DYE?

In our opinion, unless there are very good business or social reasons as in the case of actors and actresses, teachers or other business and professional men and women, it is much better to let Nature take its course and not resort to hair dyeing. Home dyeing is rarely a success, no matter how easy the manufacturers of dyes tell you it is. If you feel you must dye your hair, have the dye expertly applied by a professional so that even the most critical eye cannot detect it.

SOMETHING ELSE ABOUT HAIR DYEING

Hair dyeing is a highly specialized and dangerous branch of Beauty Culture, as is well known by every make-up department in the Film and T.V. Studios. As noted, it is seldom possible for a satisfactory job to be done at home, regardless of the claims of the dye manufacturers. Even with the best hair dyes there are problems in preventing unhealthy systemic conditions from developing. The porosity of the hair as well as the kind of dye must be calculated. Some hair absolutely refuses to "take" dye, while other hair will assume pronounced and ugly shades. Look around you and observe the horrible, harsh colors of most dyed hair.

If you are going to dye your own hair, the only sensible thing to do is to make a test first. Apply the dye to be used (following the directions that accompany it) to a small strand (from roots to end) of the underneath hair. Allow it to remain the required length of time, then wash and dry the dyed strand. If it is satisfactory, the whole head may be dyed.

In no case should dye be applied if there is any skin disease of the scalp, such as eruptions, psoriasis, eczema, etc. To be certain that your skin will not be adversely affected by the dye, wash a spot of skin behind the ear and apply some of the dye with cotton. Leave it on for a day, then remove with soap and water . . . or if it is obstinate, use peroxide or oil. If no inflammation results you are probably safe.

Never apply one make of dye over a different one. Hair breakage or extreme colors may result.

Again, it is our personal opinion that all dyes tend to make the hair dry and brittle. This condition becomes aggravated when the hair is waved or curled by means of heat. Hair dye manufacturers do not hesitate to give glib assurances that the hair may be waved or curled safely after using their products, but dyed hair is never immune from the effects of the various heating methods in general use for permanent waving. This "chamber of horrors" is not an exaggerated wax museum ... but simple scientific facts that have been concealed from the public by a mass of printed misinformation in the interests of promoting specific products.

Physicians know how widespread is the complaint of grayness. They understand the circumstances that compel men and women to want to appear young. As is the case with so many things affecting the body, *sound medical advice beforehand* may avoid much woe for those who feel they must dye their hair. It is the wise thing to do to seek your physician's advice ... and gray hairs are supposed to be a sign of wisdom. If the questionable charm of dyed or bleached hair proves too alluring and is tempting you—remember it is a calculated risk.

A SAD ADVENTURE IN HAIR DYEING

At the Los Angeles Athletic Club I had a handsome friend —a fellow member whom I will call Frank—with whom I played many competitive games of handball. Frank owned an exclusive ladies shoe store and had the best clientele in the city. The society and wealthy ladies and movie stars were all good customers of Frank's stylish shoes.

When Frank reached his early forties the gray hair started to appear at his temples, and the sight sent my friend into a panic. It became a dark cloud over his head. As his friend I tried to quiet him down. But I could not compete with the advertisements of the hair dye manufacturers who said that gray hair made one look old ... that gray hair was ugly and morbid ... and that when you were gray you were "over the hill" and life would pass you by.

My handsome friend Frank had a vivid imagination and believed that his gray hairs would lose for him his splendid lady shoe customers. In vain, I tried to tell him that he really looked more handsome and distinguished with the gray hair at his temples. But poor Frank was brainwashed into the conviction that his gray hair marked the end of life.

So Frank got his hair dyed. He went to an exclusive Men's

Hair Styling Shop in Hollywood which specialized in dyeing hair and had a professional job done on his. He was like a kid with a new toy. Now he had the "natural color" of his hair again! Every week he went faithfully to the hair dye shop for a fresh dye job. This continued for about five years. The grayer Frank's hair became, the more dye they would soak into his hair and scalp.

Things started to happen to Frank's health and appearance. Frank started to slow down physically. In time he told me that he just did not have the energy and strength to play handball with me. His skin color became sallow and pale. His eyes lost their sparkle and he no longer appeared boyish. Soon the lack of exercise made him flabby and pudgy.

Others noticed the dye job. Who said women are the only gossips? Men do their full share of gossiping, too. In the locker and cloak rooms fellow club members would comment ... "Who does Frank think he's fooling with that dye job on his hair?" ... "Frank is fooling no one with that dye on his hair—not even himself." And the truth of the matter was that anyone could plainly see that Frank's hair was dyed.

MY FRIEND IS POISONED BY HAIR DYE

Now get the picture. For five years Frank had been going every week to have his hair dyed. He had been slowly poisoned, the poison of the dye having been absorbed through the pores of the scalp and gradually distributed throughout his body by the blood stream.

The climax of this accumulated poisoning occurred one day when five of us were having lunch together at the Athletic Club. Frank was sitting across the table from me and I could study him carefully. When we sat down to lunch, his skin looked pale and greenish yellow, and I noticed that he could not focus his eyes on me. Suddenly he slumped over onto the table, completely blacked out.

Fortunately one of our luncheon companions was a doctor, and I told him what I thought was wrong with Frank.

"Paul," he said, "I know you're right. I think that Frank

has been slowly poisoned by chemical hair dye over the years."

Frank was rushed to the hospital, and for a few weeks he had a pretty rough time of it. The doctor and I told him what we thought—that all of his troubles were due to this long, slow hair dye poisoning.

Frank gave up the weekly hair dyeing routine and slowly recovered his health. It was a long hard pull, but his good doctor friend and I as nutritionist worked together to put him back on his feet. Frank's hair is entirely gray now. But to many people, including myself, he seems far more handsome with his gray hair than he did even when it was naturally brown. His business has expanded. Instead of one exclusive ladies shoe store, he now has four.

WITH TIME THERE WILL BE CHANGES IN YOUR APPEARANCE

Let us say once more that the most permanent thing in life is change. Nature changes the green leaves of summer into the many beautiful colors of autumn. And Nature changes our naturally colored hair into gray. It does not mean that you are old when this happens. It means that this permanent thing called change is operating. Why fight it? Go along with Nature!

In our work we have the opportunity of knowing many men and women who are gray, and we find that gray hair softens their features. The handsomest men and women we know—in fashionable clubs, in the entertainment world, in various businesses and professions, in all walks of life—are turning gray or are fully gray. We know many movie directors, actors, actresses and T.V. personalities who are justly proud of their gray hair.

If a man or a woman feels that dyed hair will make him or her look and feel younger and more attractive, we have nothing against it. But we do say in all sincerity that before dyeing the hair, a dermatologist should be consulted. Let this skin specialist tell you just what dye should be used on your hair and scalp. He can give you valuable professional advice that can save you from going through the same experience as my friend Frank.

SIMPLIFIED RULES FOR THE CARE OF THE HAIR

Let us now review the Program of Hair and Scalp Care which we have outlined for you in this book.

1. REMEMBER, "YOU ARE WHAT YOU EAT." The hair and scalp have to be nourished just the same as the brain, heart and every one of the billions of cells in your body. No structure is stronger than the material it is made of. As noted in this book, avoid all foodless foods. These are the foods that may produce deficiencies and build a highly toxic condition of your blood stream. Both malnutrition and toxic poisons are enemies of a good head of thick, healthy hair.

Salt and salty foods are enemies of your hair, as well as of your heart, arteries and veins.

Tea, coffee, chocolate, alcohol, cola drinks and soft drinks are foodless beverages. They contain highly toxic materials such as tannic acid, theine, caffeine and toxic acids. They contribute nothing for the good of your hair and body.

The Proteins—either animal or vegetable—are important for good, healthy hair and scalp. They are found in meats— including beef, lamb, fish and fowl, in nuts, seeds such as sunflower, pumpkins, etc., in avocados, natural cheese, raw milk, pastuerized milk, goat's milk, soya beans, soybean milk powder, legumes (dry beans of all kinds), eggs, brewer's yeast, natural brown rice, wild rice, whole grain rye, oats, millet and wheat.

Besides Protein, your hair needs Calcium, Iodine, Organic Sulphur and Silicon in a Balanced Natural Diet which also contains all the vital nutrients for complete nourishment.

(NOTE: The *Bragg Health Food Cook Books* contain pages of information and recipes that are important to every person desiring to eat for better health. See back page of this book for details.)

2. GOOD CIRCULATION IS ESSENTIAL. You must have a steady flow of well nourished blood into the hair and scalp areas, as well as plenty of oxygen. We have already

discussed the value and methods of massage. In the following section we will give you the Hair Hygiene Program used by the Hollywood Stars.

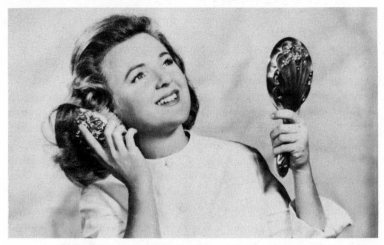

Patricia Bragg has lustrous, luxuriant hair, which she brushes 100 strokes daily. This regular brushing stimulates circulation in blood vessels closest to the hair roots, helps to distribute the natural oil of the scalp, and keeps the scalp free from accumulations of dead epidermal cells.

3.   BRUSHING THE HAIR cannot be overdone, and should be done at least twice daily.

4.   HAIR SHOULD BE THOROUGHLY WASHED twice a week, and more often if the condition of the scalp warrants it.

5.   THE BEST SHAMPOOS to use on the hair are pH balanced protein, amino acids or castile shampoos.

6.   RULES FOR THE SHAMPOO: 2 to 3 latherings of shampoo should be followed by 2 thorough rinsings in warm water, then a cold water rinse to stimulate circulation. Patricia varies the last rinse by adding sometimes apple cider vinegar, or an amino acid or protein hair conditioner, leaving on a few minutes, then rinse well. If distilled water is available (rain water is o.k.), this is perfect for final last rinse — even after protein or amino acid rinse.

7.   COMBS should have blunt, smooth teeth.

8. BRUSHES should have firm bristles of varying length to penetrate the hair. Brushes with softer bristles for purposes of glossing the hair may also be employed to advantage.

9. FOR HAIR WITH A TENDENCY TO DRYNESS: The white of an egg may be used with the first shampoo water. An hour or even the night before shampooing, almond, olive, castor or coconut oil may be rubbed into scalp and hair.

10. SEA BATHING is definitely beneficial to the hair and scalp. Rinse afterward with fresh water.

11. GO BAREHEADED WHENEVER POSSIBLE. The wind, rain, snow and sunshine stimulate your hair. You will not "catch" a cold exposing your hair and scalp to the elements. You "catch" colds at the dining-room table. A cold is Nature's way of detoxifying the body of wastes.

12. DON'T PUT VANITY ABOVE HAIR HEALTH. Some women go to the beauty shop, get their hair set—and for a week or more will give it no care or brushing because this would disturb the hairdo. This is a perfect way to bring on unhealthy conditions of the scalp and hair. It will start to drop out and become unmanageable. The scalp has to be massaged and the hair brushed daily to remain healthy and beautiful.

13. DON'T CLOG THE PORES OF YOUR SCALP. Many men clog these pores with creams and lotions—then wonder why they lose their hair. These pores must be kept clean and functioning for a healthy scalp and hair.

14. TAKE TIME TO RELAX. Even ten minutes a day on a slant board or with your back flat on the floor and legs up will stretch muscles and restore nourishing blood circulation to feed your hair and scalp.

15. PROPER QUANTITY AND QUALITY OF SLEEP is necessary for Nature to cleanse and rebuild your body after the day's activities. Get 8 hours of restful sleep every night for a healthy body, scalp and hair.

16. BEFORE YOU DYE YOUR HAIR or color it artificially, consult a dermatologist for scientific advice. It may save you a heartbreak.

TO SUM UP: Eat natural foods ... massage the temporal blood vessels. .. wash hair often and massage scalp daily ... get proper amount of relaxation and sleep ... and you will have a head of hair to be proud of.

ADDITIONAL POINTERS ON HAIR CARE

HAIR SETTING—Whether you set your hair yourself or have it done professionally, it should first be toweled almost dry by hand. Damp-dry hair takes a set as well or better than wet hair, and shortens the process considerably. Naturally wavy or curly hair can be easily finger-set into a becoming hair style. If your hair is straight, or if you feel it needs more "body" to hold the set, use a mild, non-toxic wave lotion that contains lanolin. Apply it lightly to the sections you wish to wave or curl. Never soak your hair with any wave lotion, and never apply the lotion direct to the scalp. (It is only the hair you wish to curl!) If you use curlers, never use metal ones as these tend to break the hair.

HAIR SPRAYS—are not recommended. If you feel that you must have a hair spray for special occasions, use the least toxic you can find. Many shops and stores carry anti-allergy hair preparations, and it would be wise to check these.

PERMANENTS—either the professional or the do-it-yourself variety—are harmful to the hair, because of the harsh chemicals used in nearly all permanent wave preparations. Recently a new line of "protein" permanents has come on the market, claiming to be less harmful than others. Investigate, if you feel that you must have a permanent.

BLEACHING—strips the hair and leaves it in a weakened condition. Avoid it!

HAIR TRIMMING—is generally beneficial, especially if your hair has a tendency to split at the ends. Patricia keeps her long hair full at the ends by having it trimmed about ½ inch every two or three months.

THE LONG AND THE SHORT OF IT FOR ACTIVE PEOPLE—Many active people—women as well as men, children as well as adults—prefer short hair because it can be easily shampooed daily under the shower, dries quickly and is generally more manageable for an active, outdoor life. Many women and girls, however, enjoy having long hair—and enjoy outdoor sports as well. Patricia, who has a full head of lovely, long hair, participates in all types of athletics. She keeps her hair neat and easily managed by wearing it either in a pony tail or in loose braids—not only during her outdoor activity, but also while performing household tasks. She never uses rubber bands on her hair, but recommends elasticized cord. This holds pony tails or braids firmly in place without breaking the hair. Ribbon bows or artificial flowers may be added for a festive, feminine effect.

HERE IS THE HOLLYWOOD PROGRAM FOR BEAUTIFUL HAIR

Movie Stars, T.V. Stars and Night Club Entertainers must appear before the public at their very best. Their hair must be flawlessly groomed. These people know the importance of healthy, beautiful hair, and they follow our instructions to the letter.

As we have told you in this book, you are most often judged by your personal appearance. If your hair looks like the end of a broom you have no one to blame but yourself. You must recognize that you never get anything for nothing ... and to have a head of beautiful, thick, healthy hair you must work for it. That's what the Stars of the entertainment world do.

And here is how they do it. We will now outline for you the same Hair Hygiene Program that we have outlined for the highest paid Movie Stars.

When I see fashionable tables set out in all their grandeur, I imagine gout and other ailments, lying in ambush, among the dishes.—Luigi Cornaro

GIVE YOUR HAIR PLENTY OF OXYGEN INSIDE AND OUT

Your hair and scalp thrive on oxygen. Yet nine out of ten people don't give their bodies enough oxygen. They are oxygen-starved ... simply because they don't exercise enough or breathe deeply enough.

Oxygen does these definite things: 1) Purifies and enriches the blood; 2) Aids digestion and elimination; 3) Tones up the whole system; 4) Builds resistance and power; 5) Creates strong hair, healthy scalp, bone, sinew and muscle.

Many Hollywood Stars—men and women—have luxuriant, healthy hair because they follow the Hair Hygiene Program which we recommend for them. They walk bareheaded in the sun and air, giving their bodies Nature's basic exercise and at the same time ventilating their hair and scalp.

They also follow a regular daily routine of deep breathing and scalp massage.

Remember breathing is the "stream of life." The oxygen in the air we breathe is power. Power to help in building a healthy body and a healthy scalp and a head of thick, beautiful hair.

(NOTE: The Bragg book on *Yoga Super Brain Breathing* fully explains the whys, hows, examples, etc. of deep Brain Breathing. See back pages of this book for details.)

MASSAGE YOUR SCALP IN THE PROPER POSITION

Here is how you can combine deep breathing and scalp massage for better health and more beautiful hair.

When possible do this outdoors—but if weather does not permit, open windows and stand out in the middle of the room where there is no furniture. See that there is a steady stream of fresh air circulating in the room.

Now take a full, deep breath of fresh air and hold the breath, while you bend forward from the waist with the knees bent. Get your head as near the floor as possible. You will feel a tremendous flow of oxygenated blood into all parts of the hair and scalp.

While in this position place your fingers on the side of your lower neck and gently push forward the blood of the temporal artery, as shown in the illustrations on pages 74 to 78.

As you push up and in front of your ears, release your fingers and push the palms of the hands above the eyes and across the forehead. Hold for a second the blood you have thus trapped.

Release your hands and your breath as you return to a standing position. Do this with an easy motion, not abruptly.

Repeat this procedure five to ten times.

(NOTE: We have used the words "push UP" meaning *upward toward the top of your head*, although your head is leaning downward. But to massage or push the blood "downward" would mean back toward your neck away from the scalp—which you should never do.)

TAKE IT EASY AT FIRST

After your scalp has loosened up, you may repeat this Deep Breathing and Scalp Massage Exercise as many as 30 times. But make this increase gradually. Take it easy at first.

Many of you have never massaged your scalp in the way we have found to be most beneficial. And, if you are like most people, you are likely to think that if a little massage is good, more will be better. This is not so, when you first start to massage your scalp. You must take it easy and build up gradually.

You must realize that at the beginning of this Program many of you will have scalps as tight as a drumhead. Overly vigorous massage at this time could do incalculable harm. So don't be like a personal friend of ours who did not follow our directions. He massaged his scalp too vigorously BEFORE it was sufficiently loosened, and lacerated the skin of his scalp. It took many weeks to heal and thus delayed his continuance of this Program for Hair and Scalp Health.

To demonstrate to yourself how tight your scalp is, put the palms of your hands on each side of your head near the hat line, interlock your fingers across your scalp, and very gently squeeze upward. You will probably hear tiny adhesions and flesh snapping as your scalp loosens up.

REMEMBER THE PARABLE OF THE SOWER

Remember that when you first start this Program, the hair soil on your head is probably quite thin and you must act accordingly. Overly vigorous massage and pulling at this time could cause the weaker hairs to come out. Hair needs to be anchored firmly in a thick, loose, rich hair soil fed by a healthy blood stream. Many people's hair is growing in such a haphazard manner on top of a drumhead tight scalp that care must be taken to loosen the scalp and enrich the soil, just as you would the earth when planting a garden.

Most of you remember the Parable of the Sower in the Bible (Matthew 13). Some seed fell by the wayside and the birds ate it. Some fell on stony places and the sun scorched it. Some fell in among thorns and weeds and was smothered. But other seed fell into GOOD ground and brought forth a crop— some thirtyfold, some sixtyfold and some a hundredfold. The reason these crops grew so well was because the soil was rich, deep and fertile.

Does this not teach you that a thick, rich hair soil on your head fed by a healthy blood stream could produce results similar to the seed growing in good ground?

TRY A "SCALP WARM-UP" FIRST

In addition to the Deep Breathing and Scalp Massage Exercise, many of the Hollywood personalities who consult us also use the Six Standard Massage Positions as illustrated in this book. See pages 74 to 78.

BEFORE you start this more vigorous massage, give yourself a Hair and Scalp Warm-Up.

Press the hands firmly upon the scalp and move it back and forth, up and down with a circular motion until every portion of the scalp is soft and flexible and moves freely. You may want to help soften and loosen it with the aid of a good oil such as castor oil, olive oil, etc.

As your scalp loosens, gradually go into more vigorous massage to further stimulate hair growth. The skin of the entire scalp should be manipulated. Pinching and kneading the scalp is also beneficial.

A gentle but firm pulling of the hair improves its strength and stimulates its growth. Pass the closed fingers through every portion of the hair to effect an even pulling all over the scalp.

Remember you cannot have good hair and scalp health with a tight scalp. At first your scalp will be sensitive and will hurt a little. It is very much like exercising the muscles for the first time. But this will pass. Soon you will be able to put more vigor into your scalp and hair work-out. You will be able to use the tremendous strength of the hands and fingers on your scalp and hair.

We also recommend the use of a small round plastic hair massager. Its plastic teeth help lift up dandruff, grease and other foreign matter.

FIFTEEN MINUTES A DAY THE HOLLYWOOD WAY

Your hair and your scalp are important to your wellbeing as well as to your appearance, so don't let anything stop you from your daily treatments. Being busy is no excuse. Some of the busiest people in the world always find time each day to go through this Hair Hygiene Program.

No profession is more demanding and strenuous than that of the entertainment world. Yet actors, actresses, directors and others of Motion Picture, T.V. and Night Club fame faithfully carry out the Hair Hygiene Program that we recommend.

It takes only 15 minutes of this routine to send the blood coursing into the scalp. You should do this at least once a day —several times a day is better. Once you start this scalp and hair stimulation program and discover the benefits of Deep Breathing and Scalp Massage, you will realize how foolish is the excuse that you "don't have time."

We practice what we preach. Patricia and I live as busy a life as any two humans in the world, yet we always find time to take care of our hair and scalp.

You will find it rewarding, too.

HOT OIL TREATMENT TWICE MONTHLY

Here is the second step in the Hair Hygiene Program of the Hollywood Stars who have such beautiful and luxuriant hair. This is a hot castor oil self-treatment.

Heat some castor oil to a temperature that is comfortable but stimulating to the skin of your scalp—about the same temperature of the water of a hot tub bath.

Rub the heated castor oil thoroughly into the hair and scalp. Then apply very hot damp towels around the entire head to steam the oil into hair and scalp. Continue the hot towel treatment for at least ten minutes.

Allow the oil to remain on the scalp and hair for at least another 20 minutes. Some Hollywood Stars leave the oil on overnight, wrapping the head with a large, dry turkish towel.

Then remove the oil with a vigorous shampoo—following our previous instruction (See pages 55, 56). Remember to scrub the scalp with your fingers to help remove all dirt, grease and dandruff which have been loosened by the hot oil treatment, and rinse the hair and scalp thoroughly, finishing off with a vinegar or lemon juice rinse followed by cold water. Dry the hair thoroughly with towels by hand and preferably in the sun. Do not use artificial heat unless absolutely necessary.

This Hot Oil Self-Treatment should be done twice a month. In time, along with your daily Hair and Scalp program, you will see remarkable changes for the better in the health of your hair and your scalp.

EVERY DAY OF YOUR LIFE GET EVERY
DEAD HAIR OUT OF YOUR HEAD

To have healthy, luxuriant hair you must follow this firm rule every day of your life. This is a very important part of your Hair Hygiene Program. When you allow dead hair to remain in the head you start to have hair and scalp problems. New hair finds it difficult to come in when it is blocked by a dead hair.

The pulling of the hair and the vigorous massage, as we have instructed you previously, loosens the dead hairs from your head. Out they come, and in their place starts to grow strong new hair.

Brushing and combing must be combined with massaging and pulling to remove all the dead hairs. Remember you have thousands of hairs on your head, and as old hairs complete their lifespan and die, new hairs are ready to replace them. This is occurring all the time. By getting rid of the dead hairs you help to insure a strong new growth.

You should have at least two sets of brushes—one very stiff for the first vigorous brushing, and one softer for the polishing process. And remember that the best position for brushing your hair is with the head forward and downward below the heart level, feet apart and knees slightly bent.

Now you can see how all phases of this Hair Hygiene Program are coordinated. First to feed your blood stream with the essential nutrients ... then to feed it oxygen and stimulate circulation by deep breathing and scalp massage ... cleansing with the hot oil treatment and proper shampooing ... brushing and combing to remove dead hairs and cultivate luxuriant new growth ... and don't forget relaxation and sleep, the healthfully restorative beautifiers.

CHOOSE A BECOMING HAIR STYLE— AND YOU'RE ALWAYS IN STYLE

Remember, most people judge you by your looks ... and your hair is the key to your appearance. It is the mirror of your health ... and your health greatly influences your personality. So judgment by appearance has its basis in logic, after all.

There is wisdom in the folk saying that, "If the bed is made, the house looks tidy; and if your hair is neat, you look well dressed."

Of first importance, of course, is carrying out this Program of Hair and Scalp Health. Now, take full advantage of your beautiful, healthy hair by arranging it in the most becoming fashion. Don't defeat your whole purpose by falling for a faddish hair style that is unbecoming.

Again take a tip from the glamorous Hollywood Stars, women and men. They must always look their best. Not only do they follow a healthful Hair Hygiene Program . . . but they make sure that their hair is dressed in the manner most becoming and best suited to their individual personalities. And they always look in style.

This does not mean that you should copy your favorite star's hairdo. It may not be becoming to you. Study yourself, your face, the shape of your head, your figure . . . and your personality. "Know thyself." Then—with expert help if necessary—choose a simple, natural style of hairdressing that is distinctively YOURS, expressive of YOU. If you do this wisely, you will always look smart and fashionable—no matter what the latest current fad may be. *The keynote is always to be natural!* A *naturally* becoming hair style is the crowning touch to your "Crowning Glory."

SPECIAL NOTE TO MEN—A full, fluffy, natural head of hair is not only healthier but far more becoming to every man than hair that is slicked back and plastered down with gooey pomades. Soft, wavy hair that is clean and well groomed can make a homely man appear goodlooking, and make a handsome man even more so. Don't allow your hair to be cut too short—and always leave it full over the ears, to avoid that "big-ear look." Take a tip from Hollywood Actors who use a mild non-toxic wave lotion that contains lanolin. Apply this lightly to the hair while it is damp-dry and push in a wave with your fingers, allow to dry and then comb. The result is a wave that looks natural and stays in.

YOU HAVE JOINED FORCES WITH MOTHER NATURE FOR LUXURIANT HAIR

As you see—from beginning to finale—this Natural Program of Hair Culture is using all the forces of Nature to help you have beautiful, luxuriant hair and a healthy scalp.

Life is largely a matter of chemistry.—William J. Mayo, M.D.

Your Natural Diet with all essential nutrients including Protein, Calcium, Silicon, Organic Sulphur and Iodine is contributing toward better constitutional health, the basis of Hair and Scalp Health.

Your Deep Breathing is sending large amounts of life giving oxygen through the blood stream into your hair and scalp.

By Scalp Massage and Brushing—always in the proper forward leaning position—you are stimulating circulation that helps to enrich your hair soil, and stimulating hair growth by removing dead hairs and dirt. The cleansing process is completed by Hot Oil Treatments and Proper Shampooing.

By healthful Relaxation and Restful Sleep, you are giving Mother Nature her needed opportunity for inner cleansing and restoring of your entire body.

Now that you have joined forces with Mother Nature, every step in this Program will be a joyous event. You will feel the clean, nourishing blood coursing through your body into your hair and scalp, making it tingle and feel alive. And when your hair and scalp feel buoyantly alive, so do you!

DON'T BE IMPATIENT WITH NATURE!

Don't expect miracles overnight. Remember that it takes a long time for the hair and scalp to get into an unhealthy condition ... and it will take time to return to normal, natural health. This Program of Hair and Scalp Health has helped thousands, and it will also help YOU—if you will give it time. You cannot rush Mother Nature.

The average person takes their hair for granted. They shampoo it occasionally, and they may even give it a few seconds of brushing. But that is about all the care the average hair and scalp gets. Then something tragic happens. The hair starts falling out by the handfuls, and the scalp is in an extremely unhealthy condition. Why? Simply because the average person has not followed a sensible and natural Hair Hygiene Program.

Luxuriant hair is Mother Nature's Gift to Humanity, which millions throw away because they do not know the simple

Natural Laws for Hair Hygiene. This Hair Hygiene Program will be of priceless value to you. There is no necessity for the hair to get thin and ugly. A reasonable amount of proper care will keep it strong and healthy throughout life. And if it is already falling out the same care may aid in restoring it. This Hair Hygiene Program tells the simple natural and effective methods for treating the hair and scalp—of equal benefit to men and women.

Healthy hair and a healthy scalp are important both to your appearance and your wellbeing. It gives one confidence to look into the mirror and see a full head of healthy, luxuriant hair.

The great Film Stars find it rewarding to follow this Natural Program of Hair Hygiene. And so will you. Start today on this Program and see how very satisfying it can be to you. Make this Program part of your daily life.

WORK AND LIVE THE GOOD LIFE

If there is anything we enjoy most it must be to condition our bodies to a high rate of efficiency. Once you get into this Hair and Scalp Program you will become excited and begin to take better care of your body as you see your hair and scalp improve. *Life is joyful when lived correctly.*

Remember, only YOU can cause things to happen in your life. Make things happen—don't let circumstances happen to you! YOU are the Captain of your life! You must decide what is good for you! Don't listen to negative people. All of us have had to fight this all of our lives—even within our own families. And sad to say, all those scorners are GONE! That's what following their own negative advice brought upon them.

Yes, sometimes people in your own household can become your worst ENEMY when it comes to the health life. So follow what you know is right! You are an individual and must chart YOUR OWN COURSE in life. Listen to people who have an interest in you as a human being. Live life to the fullest! Cheat the early grim reaper and undertaker—and live a long, active life. YOU CAN DO IT!

Life and living are work so you have to work at them—that's the fun of it. You don't get something for nothing and enjoy it as much as when you WORK for it! Work strengthens. Remember that! So work hard and faithfully every day at your Hair and Scalp Health Program. This is the kind of work that brings a flashing, vibrant light to the eyes and adds joy to life—so, WORK!

KNOW THY BODY

Socrates, one of the world's greatest philosophers, always urged his disciples, "Know Thyself." This is excellent philosophy. Applied to the problems of Hair and Scalp Health, it might be restated as, "Know Thy Body" and "Know Thy Hair and Scalp."

Do you know as much about your body as you do about your automobile? I'll bet you don't—and if you do, you're one person in ten thousand. Which is more valuable to you, your body or your automobile? Your body, of course! You can purchase another car, but there are no new living bodies for sale—the one you have now is your first and your last.

A car is made through and by the intelligence of man. The manufacturer, knowing man's frailty, issues a catalog in which every part of the car is described in words and pictures. He also furnishes a book of instructions on its care, and specifies the best type of fuel and oil to use. The purchaser acquires the car with what we call money, and because of its monetary value usually takes good care of it.

One's body—and that includes your hair and scalp—was not purchased with money and has no monetary value except through its earning capacity. Evolved by Nature, it is a machine which will never be even remotely approached by any manmade product in intricate mechanism, delicacy of operation and range of function. Yet its care is simple—and that again goes for the hair and scalp—based on just one rule: *Obedience to Nature's Laws.*

The chemistry of the food a person eats becomes his own body chemistry.

104

A PERSONAL MESSAGE TO THOSE WHOSE HAIR IS TURNING GRAY AND TO THOSE GETTING BALD

We have no cures for gray hair, nor have we a cure for people who are going bald or who are already bald. Our work is PREVENTION. We try with all our might to impress upon people that there are no miracles for turning gray hair back to normal nor a cure for baldness. We want that definitely understood.

From this Program of Hair and Scalp Culture, however, we have had many unsolicited testimonials from people who were turning gray and found that their hair was returning to its natural color ... and we have had people who were bald tell us that new hair was growing where there was none. We have no way to verify these testimonials, as our health students are scattered over the four corners of the world.

As we herewith state, we are not looking for cures because we have none to offer. We are strictly interested in a Program of Prevention!

The human body is self-healing and self-repairing. The recuperative powers of the body are tremendous. If you work closely with these wonderful powers of Nature—who knows what may happen to YOU!

As your instructors, we want to help YOU to HELP YOURSELF! We can go no further than to give you what is, in our opinion, the best Natural and Scientific Course in Hair Culture and Scalp Care in the world.

I am a great-grandfather and a man who has lived three-score years and ten plus—and I have one of the strongest heads of hair in the world. I owe my powerful head of thick hair to this Natural System of Hair Culture and Scalp Care. As I told you earlier in this book I had serious hair and scalp problems to overcome.

Patricia, my daughter and co-author of this book, has a beautiful head of thick, luxuriant hair with that soft, glossy, well groomed appearance.

We show by precept and example that the Hair Culture Program we are teaching you has given us tremendous benefits.

Regardless of how hopeless your hair and scalp condition may seem, you are now going to join forces with NATURE for the attainment of rewarding goals. Put your heart and your enthusiasm into this Natural Program of Hair Culture and Scalp Health.

Carry the mental picture as you work on your scalp ... that you are going to have LUXURIANT HAIR. Your mind has a tremendous influence on your body. By this Natural Method of Hair Culture you awaken, vitalize and energize the scalp, making and keeping it soft, flexible and healthy.

"VANITY"—THY NAME IS MAN

It is perfectly natural for us to be vain, for the world judges us by our personal appearance ... so it is natural for us to want and try to look our very best. But we must not let the manufacturers of wigs, toupees and hair dyes brainwash us into believing that the only people who are goodlooking are those whose heads are covered with hair that is not gray.

Remember that people who judge us on just a glance are not qualified to pass judgment upon us. This is merely a superficial judgment. We must judge others and ourselves for the total person.

We'll admit that we must all try to look our very best at all times. It gives us more confidence in ourselves and we become more attractive to others.

That is the reason we have written this book for you! So that you can do the very best with what you have. You can do no more. Because you are bald or gray, do not let this in any way give you an inferiority complex. The hair and scalp form an important part of the human body, that is true. Our advice, we repeat, is to do the very best with what you have. In working for healthy hair and scalp you will most assuredly attain better overall health. And after all, "YOUR HEALTH IS YOUR GREATEST WEALTH." Good health makes up for everything else we may lack, for with good health we are happy people. And what greater treasures are there than health and happiness!

106

SPECIAL NEW INFORMATION

In response to the many inquiries which we have received on our worldwide lecture tours and through the mail, we are adding this Special Supplement to the Second Edition of "YOUR HEALTH AND YOUR HAIR" . . . giving you a detailed chart of **Vitamins and Minerals Essential to Hair and Scalp Health.**

WHAT ARE VITAMINS

Most people in civilized countries today know that vitamins are important to health . . . but have only vague ideas as to why we need them and how they help us. The average person believes that a supplement of synthetic vitamins is all that is necessary. This is far from the truth. The "foodless foods" from supermarket shelves cannot be magically changed into natural nourishment simply by taking artificial vitamins. In fact, this is adding insult to injury.

Just as your diet should consist of natural "live" foods, so should your vitamin supplements come from the same source. Unfortunately, under "civilized" marketing conditions, it is impossible to obtain 100% natural foods all the time. Vitamin supplements have therefore become necessary . . . but these, too, must be derived from a **natural, organic source,** such as the Vitamin Supplements which you find in your Health Food Store.

Vitamins are not foods . . . they are accessory food **substances** . . . which work with other nutritional substances to carry on the life processes of the body. Vitamins help the body to assimilate food . . . rebuild tissues . . . resist disease . . . insure proper growth. They aid in almost all physical and mental functions.

Vitamins are not manufactured by the human body . . . we must get them from the food we eat. And we must have a steady intake of these vital vitamins, because they are not stored by the body. We do not get them, however, from our usual diet of modern civilization . . . vitamins are volatile, and are easily destroyed by heat, oxidation and processing.

Hair Health is Related Both Directly and Indirectly to Your Vitamin Intake

Some vitamins influence directly the growth and condition of the hair . . . others influence it indirectly in relation to the general health of the body, which is always reflected in hair and scalp conditions. Let's review these essential vitamins and their functions.

VITAMIN A

Hair and Scalp Health are directly affected by Vitamin A. A deficiency of this important vitamin can result in drying and clogging of the sebaceous glands, which supply oil to the hair and scalp. Dry, coarse hair, dry scalp and loss of hair are the results.

So be sure to get your quota of Vitamin A for lustrous, healthy hair! The standard daily requirement is 5,000 international units . . . and some authorities advise up to 50,000 i.u.'s per day for extreme cases of deficiency.

Vitamin A is also essential for healthy skin and nails . . . for strong eyesight . . . normal growth and reproduction . . . and as a protection against ear and nasal infections and kidney stones.

Sources of Vitamin A . . . The prime source is cod or halibut liver oil, which may be obtained in either tablet or liquid form. Food sources include liver and desicated (dried and powdered) liver . . . carrots . . . spinach, lettuce, broccoli, dandelion greens and other green leafy vegetables . . . egg yolk (fertile) . . . and whole milk.

THE B COMPLEX VITAMINS

Hair growth and color are affected by the B Complex or "family" of vitamins, both individually and interdependently. Several are directly related to hair health . . . others indirectly in relation to general health, especially of the nervous system. All vitamins in the B Complex should be included in the daily diet.

108

Sources of B Complex . . . Prime sources are brewers yeast and liver (whole and desicated). Plain, natural yogurt is also considered to include the entire B Complex. Other foods which contain many of the B Complex Vitamins are natural cheese . . . egg yolk (fertile) . . . fish, kidneys, lean meat . . . soybeans, sunflower seeds . . . wheat germ, whole grains . . . fresh fruit.

Individual Members of the B Complex "Family" include:

Vitamin B-1 (Thiamine) . . . This vitamin is essential for life itself. It helps to transport oxygen to all the cells of the body . . . to convert glucose into energy . . . to maintain the health of the nervous system. Varying degrees of deficiency are evidenced in symptoms ranging from fatigue to mental disturbance. **Sources** include brewers yeast, liver (whole and desicated), blackstrap molasses, egg, powdered milk, wheat germ, rice polishings, yogurt. Secondary sources are raw nuts, peas, sunflower seeds, soybeans, lean meat.

Vitamin B-2 (Riboflavin) is related to Vitamin A and has similar functions . . . a deficiency can result in dry, lustreless hair. Vitamin B-2 is essential in the assimilation of proteins, the body's "building blocks" . . . and aids in maintenance of the nervous system . . . as well as in eyesight and skin condition. **Sources** include brewers yeast, liver (whole and desicated), eggs, powdered skim milk, kidneys, soybeans, peas, green leafy vegetables.

Niacin is important in the general health of the body . . . an essential in the enzyme system in making food available for energy . . . in defense against pellagra and also against anxiety and nervous tension. **Sources** are brewers yeast, liver (whole and desicated), lean meats, poultry, fish, beef heart . . . whole grains and peanuts.

Vitamin B-6 (Pyridoxine) is directly related to Hair Health . . . because of its function in utilizing amino acids in forming new protein tissue . . . and its assistance in the utilization of unsaturated fatty acids, thus preventing excessive oiliness of the scalp. **Sources** are brewers yeast, liver (whole and desicated), lean meat . . . whole grains, natural rice . . . fresh vegetables.

Inositol has a direct relationship to hair growth and color . . . and has proved a great help in cases of hair restoration. Although it cannot be considered a cure for baldness, there seems to be a definite connection between Inositol and normal hair growth. **If you have abnormal loss of hair, a supplement of pure, organic, concentrated Inositol is recommended** . . . 6 tablets of 250 mg. daily, or more in severe cases. Most **natural food sources** which contain the other B Vitamins are also good sources of Inositol.

Pantothenic Acid and Para-Amino-Benzoic Acid (PABA) . . . These two B Vitamins work together for Hair Health . . . especially in **preventing grayness** or loss of color. Experiments show that a deficiency of either one will produce the same result . . . a loss of color . . . brittleness and dryness . . . and eventually loss of hair. **Sources** include blackstrap molasses, brewers yeast, liver (whole and desicated), lean meat, broccoli, corn, eggs (fertile), potatoes, whole grains, wheat germ.

Vitamin B-12 is highly important in preventing anemia . . . and even slight anemia can result in an unhealthy condition of the hair. **Sources** are primarily beef liver (whole and desicated) and kidneys. Other good sources include brewers yeast, lean meat, eggs (fertile), whole milk, natural cheese and wheat germ.

Other B Vitamins include biotin, choline and folic acid. Folic acid has been demonstrated to have an effect on hair color. It is important, of course, to include all the B Vitamins in the diet, as their effects are inter-related.

VITAMIN C

This vital Vitamin C provides collagen . . . the substance which holds together the cells in all tissues of the body, including the hair. It is also important in many other ways . . . including functioning of the adrenal glands . . . bone formation . . . defense against infection.

Since all commercial food processing and canning destroys large amounts of Vitamin C, we must fill the body's natural need for this essential vitamin with natural, concentrated Vitamin C Supplements. **The minimum daily requirement** for an adult has been set at 60 milligrams by the Food & Nutrition Board of the National Research Council . . . but in actual practice, most authorities recommend as high as 300 mg. or more.

Rose hips are the best natural source . . . and are available in tablet, powder or liquid form. **Other sources** are fresh citrus fruits and juices . . . apples . . . cantaloupe. Vitamin C is also found, in a fair amount, in other fresh fruits and in most fresh vegetables.

VITAMIN D

Strong bones and teeth depend upon Vitamin D, which is essential for the proper utilization and assimilation of the calcium and phosphorous in the body. Although there are traces of calcium in the hair, it has not been determined whether or not Vitamin D is essential in forming hair cells.

However, **the best source** of Vitamin D . . . **sunshine** . . . has a very beneficial effect on the hair. The only good food source is fish liver oil, especially cod and halibut . . . these tablets provide the natural requirement for both Vitamins A and D.

VITAMIN E

Vitamin E is directly related to Hair and Scalp Health . . . as it assists the body in utilizing unsaturated fatty acids, important in the natural oil of the scalp (sebum). Vitamin E is also essential in human reproduction . . . muscular tone, including the heart . . . healing of wounds and infections.

Prime source is wheat germ. Since this essential element is removed from commercial, refined flours, it must be provided by a food supplement. Both wheat germ and wheat germ oil may be obtained at your Health Food Store. Other whole grains, whole cereals, vegetable oils also contain E.

ORGANIC MINERALS

So many people think of minerals only as those which come directly from the earth . . . inorganic minerals . . . that I must stress the fact that the minerals which are so important to the human body have undergone a change into an organic state. Only plants can assimilate inorganic minerals from the soil. By the process of photosynthesis, plants change these inorganic minerals into organic minerals, which can be assimilated by animals, including the human. So, when you buy Mineral Supplements, be sure that these are derived from plant or animal sources — not directly from the earth. You can no more digest inorganic minerals than you can dirt.

Let it be understood, then, that all minerals referred to in this book are organic minerals. They are essential to the body, even in trace amounts . . . vital to cell reproduction and the assimilation and utilization of other food elements and substances. They are present in all body tissues, including hair.

MINERALS IMPORTANT TO HEALTHY HAIR

The health of your hair and scalp are definitely affected by the minerals which are integral elements of these tissues . . . and also by others which help regulate the general overall health of the body. The most important are discussed here.

Calcium is needed by the human body in greater amounts than any other mineral. Although most of it is found in the bones and teeth, calcium is essential to the proper functioning of the parathyroid glands which are important in hair growth. For proper assimilation of calcium by the body tissues, phosphorous and Vitamin D must also be present. **The best supplementary source of calcium is bone meal,** because it also contains the correct balance of phosphorous and Vitamin D. **Food sources** include raw certified or powdered skim milk, sea kelp, blackstrap molasses, fertile eggs, natural cheese, yogurt and fresh fruit.

Phosphorous is also required in large amounts by the body. It is essential in the formation of new tissue, including hair. **Sources** include bone meal as a supplement, and all protein foods.

Chlorine is a digestion aid and a cleanser of toxic wastes from body cells. Laboratory experiments have shown that even a small chlorine deficiency results in loss of hair by animals . . . and there is a definite possibility that the same may be true with humans. **Sources** are sea kelp, dulse, leafy greens, milk and tomatoes.

Iodine . . . As previously discussed (page 29), iodine is indispensable to the health of the hair as well as the rest of the body. It is essential to the functioning of the thyroid gland, which regulates body metabolism, circulation, resistance to disease, mental development. Iodine deficiency affects the hair by causing it to fall out, turn gray prematurely, become brittle and lustreless. **Best supplementary source is sea kelp**, either in tablet form (5-grain recommended) or in powdered form, used as seasoning. Dulse is also a good source. **All sea food** contains organic iodine.

Potassium affects hair growth because of its function in the utilization of protein, so essential in hair and scalp health (see page 25). Potassium is also particularly important for health of the heart. **Sources** include sea kelp, dulse, blackstrap molasses, potatoes, carrots, leafy green vegetables, whole grains, fruit (especially bananas) and honey.

Silicon is one of the trace minerals necessary for healthy hair. It works in conjunction with Vitamin A. **Sources** are steel cut oatmeal, oat-straw tea, fresh carrot and tomato juice, brewers yeast, sea kelp, liver (whole and desicated).

Secondary sources include other oat and whole grain products, fertile eggs, fish, lean meat, raw nuts and seeds, carob powder.

Magnesium, although found principally in bone tissue, has numerous functions . . . including aid in blood circulation. A magnesium deficiency restricts blood vessel activity . . . and can be first evidenced in the scalp, where the circulation is probably the most difficult in the body to maintain. **Sources** include bone meal, sea kelp, blackstrap molasses, sunflower seeds and wheat germ. Magnesium is also found in fertile egg yolk, milk, cucumbers, celery, whole grains and citrus fruits.

Sodium is an integral part of the hair, essential in protein synthesis and also an aid in the assimilation of other minerals. **Sources** include all fresh vegetables and lean meats, as well as seafood and sea kelp. IMPORTANT NOTE: Remember that it is organic sodium which your body needs . . . **not inorganic as in table salt** (sodium chloride). **Do not use salt!** . . . your body cannot digest it . . . it overloads your kidneys . . . and waterlogs your tissues. Throw your salt shaker away . . . or fill it with powdered sea kelp!

Iron is essential in the formation of hemoglobin, the red substance in your blood which carries life-giving oxygen to all the cells of your body, including your hair and scalp. A deficiency in iron produces anemia, which directly affects the hair by causing it to become dry and lustreless. **Sources** of organic iron are blackstrap molasses and liver (whole and desicated) . . . also brewers yeast, fertile egg yolks, soybeans, wheat germ, green leafy vegetables, peanuts, all fresh fruits.

Sulphur is the integral element of the hair cell which gives the hair its sheen and lustre. Approximately 5% of the hair is composed of sulphur . . . which is a protein compound, occurring primarily in the amino acids cystine and methionine. If your hair is lifeless and dull, your system is no doubt deficient in sulphur. **Prime source is a raw, fresh, fertile egg daily**. Other sources are fish, carrots, cabbage, brussel sprouts, honey and most protein foods.

114

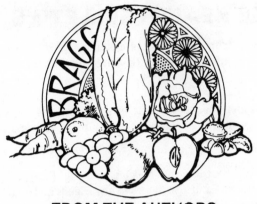

FROM THE AUTHORS

This book was written for YOU. It can be your passport to the Good Life. We Professional Nutritionists join hands in one common objective — a high standard of health for all and many added years to your life. Scientific Nutrition points the way — Nature's Way — the only lasting way to build a body free of degenerative diseases and premature aging. This book teaches you how to work with Nature and not against her. Doctors, dentists, and others who care for the sick, try to repair depleted tissues which too often mend poorly if at all. Many of them praise the spreading of this new scientific message of natural foods and methods for long-lasting health and youthfulness at any age. To speed the spreading of this tremendous message, this book was written.

Statements in this book are recitals of scientific findings, known facts of physiology, biological therapeutics, and reference to ancient writings as they are found. Paul C. Bragg has been practicing the natural methods of living for over 70 years, with highly beneficial results, knowing they are safe and of great value to others, and his daughter Patricia Bragg works with him to carry on the Health Crusade. They make no claims as to what the methods cited in this book will do for one in any given situation, and assume no obligation because of opinions expressed.

No cure for disease is offered in this book. No foods or diets are offered for the treatment or cure of any specific ailment. Nor is it intended as, or to be used as, literature for any food product. Paul C. Bragg and Patricia Bragg express their opinions solely as Public Health Educators, Professional Nutritionists and Teachers.

Certain persons considered experts may disagree with one or more statements in this book, as the same relate to various nutritional recommendations. However, any such statements are considered, nevertheless, to be factual, as based upon long-time experience of Paul C. Bragg and Patricia Bragg in the field of human health.

SEND FOR IMPORTANT
FREE HEALTH BULLETINS

Patricia Bragg, from time to time sends News Bulletins on latest Health and Nutrition Discoveries. These are sent *free of charge!*

The Health Builder, the magazine devoted to Nutrition and Physical Fitness, is also sent *free* to those who are interested in gaining and maintaining superb health!

If you wish to receive these *free bulletins* and The Health Builder— please send your name and also names of any friends and relatives you wish, using reverse side.

HEALTH SCIENCE Box 7, Santa Barbara, California 93102 U.S.A.

name   (please print)

address

city   state   zip code

name   (please print)

address

city   state   zip code

name   (please print)

address

city   state   zip code

PLEASE CUT ALONG DOTTED LINE

Please send Free Health Bulletins to these friends and relatives:

Name
_____

Address
_____

City _____ State _____ Zip Code _____

. . . .

Name
_____

Address
_____

City _____ State _____ Zip Code _____

. . . .

Name
_____

Address
_____

City _____ State _____ Zip Code _____

. . . .

Name
_____

Address
_____

City _____ State _____ Zip Code _____

. . . .

Name
_____

Address
_____

City _____ State _____ Zip Code _____

. . . .

Name
_____

Address
_____

City _____ State _____ Zip Code _____

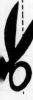

BRAGG
Live Longer, Live Stronger
Self-Improvement
LIBRARY

Let These Amazing Health Books Show You, Your Family
And Friends The Road To Health, Happiness And A Long,
Vital Life! Each Of These Books Is A Priceless And Valuable
Treasure To Help Safeguard Your Health.

PATRICIA BRAGG, Ph.D.

Nutritionist, Beauty and Health Consultant

Advisor to World Leaders, Glamorous Hollywood Stars,
Singers, Dancers, Athletes

LECTURER and AUTHOR

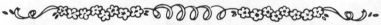

Daughter of the world renowned health authority, Paul C. Bragg, Patricia Bragg has won international fame on her own in this field. She conducts Health and Fitness Seminars for women's, men's, youth and church groups throughout the United States ... and is co-lecturer with Paul C. Bragg on tours throughout the English speaking world. Consultants to Presidents and Royalty, to Stars of Stage, Screen and TV, and to Champion Athletes, Patricia Bragg and her father are authors and co-authors of the Bragg Health Library of instructive, inspiring books.

Patricia Bragg herself is the symbol of perpetual youth, a living and sparkling example of hers and her father's precepts.

A fifth generation Californian on her mother's side, Patricia Bragg was reared by the Natural Health Method from infancy. In school, she not only excelled in athletics but also won high honors in her studies and her counseling. She is an accomplished musician and dancer ... as well as tennis player, swimmer and mountain climber ... and the youngest woman ever to be granted a U.S. Patent. An alumna of the University of California, and recently earning a Ph.D. in Health Sciences, Patricia Bragg is a popular and gifted Health Teacher.

She has been Health Consultant to that great walker, President Harry S. Truman, and to the British Royal Family.

Betty Cuthbert, Australia's "Golden Girl" who holds 16 world's records and 4 Olympic gold medals in women's track, follows Patricia Bragg's guidance. Among those who come to Patricia Bragg for advice are Clint and Maggie Eastwood, Connie Haines, Pamela Mason, Joe Feeney (singing star of Lawrence Welk's TV show) and his family of nine children, and Marilyn Van Derbur, the former Miss America who is now a famous TV personality, speaker and teacher. Patricia Bragg has helped many other official "Miss and Mr. Americas" ... plus many thousands of unofficial Mr. and Ms. Americas and their families who read her books and attend her lectures.

Life cannot be maintained unless life be taken in, and this is best done by making at least 60 percent of your diet raw and cooked vegetables, with a plentiful supply of fresh juicy fruits.

—Patricia Bragg

Jesus said: "Thy faith hath made thee whole, and go and sin no more." And that means your dietetic sins. He himself, through fasting and prayer, was able to heal the sick and cure all manner of diseases.